THIRTY DAYS

Note to the reader: Those with health problems are advised to seek the guidance of a qualified medical or psychological professional in addition to qualified macrobiotic teacher before implementing any of the dietary or other approaches presented in this book. It is essential that any reader who has any reason to suspect serious illness seek appropriate medical, nutritional or psychological advice promptly. Neither this nor any other related book should be used as a substitute for qualified care or treatment.

Published by JAPAN PUBLICATIONS, INC., Tokyo and New York

Distributors:
UNITED STATES: *Kodansha America, Inc., through Farrar, Straus & Giroux, 19 Union Square West, New York, 10003.* CANADA: *Fitzhenry & Whiteside Ltd., 195 Allstate Parkway, Markham, Ontario, L3R 4T8.* BRITISH ISLES AND EUROPEAN CONTINENT: *Premier Book Marketing Ltd., 1 Gower Street, London WC1E 6HA.* AUSTRALIA AND NEW ZEALAND: *Bookwise International, 54 Crittenden Road, Findon, South Australia 5023.* THE FAR EAST AND JAPAN: *Japan Publications Trading Co., Ltd., 1-2-1, Sarugaku-cho, Chiyoda-ku, Tokyo 101.*

First edition: July 1991

LCCC No. 89-63234
ISBN 0-87040-790-2

Printed in U.S.A.

THIRTY DAYS

A Program to Lower Cholesterol,
Achieve Optimal Weight, and
Prevent Serious Disease

By Aveline Kushi
and Tom Monte

Japan Publications, Inc.

Foreword

In his book, *On the Shoulders of Giants*, Columbia University professor Robert K. Merton showed that all important discoveries are made by more than one person at the same time, each working independently of the others.

A corollary to that idea is that all important advances are built upon each other. One person discovers something significant and promotes his ideas, which in turn creates a chain reaction of new advances. The most recent discovery in any field arrives like an apple in the summer, after many years in which a tree matures and finally produces fruit.

We humans are really a community of people creating an atmosphere of ideas that nourish this and succeeding generations. Discoveries do not simply happen to one person, nor do they arrive out of the blue. As the Preacher says, nothing is new under the sun.

We tend to forget this axiom. But even worse, we often forget the people who made the new discovery possible.

Nowhere is this better demonstrated than in the relationship between diet and health, and particularly in the realm of heart disease research.

Much is being made today about Dr. Dean Ornish's landmark study in which he demonstrated that coronary heart disease —the number one human killer—is reversible through a low fat and low cholesterol diet. Ornish, head of the Preventive Medicine Research Institute in Sausalito, California, has been featured in major newspapers and magazines around the country since his study was published in *Lancet*, the British medical journal, back in the summer of 1990. This was important research because no one had conducted the final scientific study that proved that heart disease could be reversed by diet alone. Ornish deserves much praise for his work, and he is getting it. In fact, his study is eclipsing all that has come before it, which, in this case, is like adding a new room to a house and making such a show of the addition that you forget the house itself.

Ornish's study came at a time when most cardiovascular disease experts already knew that diet reversed heart disease. They just did not have the study to prove it beyond the final doubt—a doubt that, in this case, was already pretty small. The scientific evidence has been pointing to this conclusion for the past forty years. Now, medical doctors who had been refusing to recommend diet as a therapy can shake their heads knowingly and say, yes, the final proof is in; we can now begin to advise diet as a means of treatment for heart disease.

We can only speculate on how the medical profession itself rationalizes its failure to recommend diet to the one million people who died annually from cardiovascular disease for the past four or five decades.

The question of how much proof is actually needed before physicians start making recommendations is an important one. It was considered extensively in a paper written in 1977 by Dr. Jeremiah Stamler, a leading cardiovascular disease researcher at Northwestern University Medical School, in Chicago, Illinois.

After examining all the important research relating diet to heart disease, much of which was done in the 1950s, Stamler concluded that if the same burden of proof were applied to other fields, we would have to place many of our most important discoveries in the realm of *hypothesis*—which amounts to little more than conjecture—rather than in the solidly established realm of *theory*, which is "a more or less verified or established explanation accounting for known fact," wrote Stamler. If the same burden of proof were placed on other disciplines, said Stamler, it would be "the hypothesis of gravity, not the theory of gravity; the hypothesis of relativity, not the theory of relativity; the hypothesis of evolution; not the theory of evolution."

That was twenty-three years ago, and now suddenly there is a new study and "final proof."

The question is this: Whose interests were being guarded in the quest for final proof: sick people or the medical profession?

In 1955, Nathan Pritikin, an inventor and engineer, con-

tracted heart disease. Two years later, he was told by his physicians that at the age of forty-two he would have to retire from
active life. His disease, they said, might bring about a fatal
heart attack if he stressed his heart during the normal demands
of work. One can only wonder how many people were given
that same advice and followed it. Fortunately, Nathan did not.

For the next ten years, Pritikin studied his own body and the
scientific research that did exist linking diet and health. From
this information, he created a diet and exercise program that
treated heart disease.

Nathan was not a college graduate; he dropped out of the
University of Chicago after finishing his sophomore year. He
was self-taught in many areas of science. Nevertheless, he created
a program that cured himself of heart disease. As impressive as
that accomplishment may have been, it was just the beginning.

Pritikin opened the Pritikin Longevity Center in 1976 and used
diet and exercise to heal tens of thousands of people of heart
disease, diabetes, arthritis, high blood pressure, and other degenerative diseases. Many of those who came to the Longevity
Center had been scheduled for by-pass surgery just before ar-
riving. Others came in wheelchairs, some in stretchers.

The vast majority of these people—even the worst among
them—left the center walking and, indeed, running. In the space
of a single month, these people were "returned to normal function," as Pritikin used to put it.

Nathan was criticized vehemently for saying that those who
stayed on his diet actually experienced reversal of coronary heart
disease. He had derived this conclusion from the vast amount
of research done on monkeys, which have similar cardiovascular
systems as humans and respond almost identically to fat and
cholesterol as humans. The studies on monkeys had demonstrated reversal. In order to reduce the heat of criticism, Nathan
backed off his claim of reversal, and instead said that people experienced return of normal function, meaning that they could
behave as if they had no disease at all.

Nathan's exhaustive research and great intellect enabled him
to understand and even master other areas of research, including

those of cancer, diabetes, and liver and kidney disease. He discovered that the scientific evidence linked these illnesses to diet, as well.

For ten years, Pritikin carried on a vociferous battle with the medical establishment, until his death in 1985. At times, his enemies used a variety of means to silence him, none of which worked. He kept on hammering out a simple yet profound message: that diet is both the cause and the cure of coronary heart disease, cancer, diabetes, and other degenerative illnesses. In the process, he forced the medical and scientific communities to wrestle with this fact, which ultimately resulted in Dean Ornish's study.

The stories of George Ohsawa and Michio Kushi are quite different from that of Pritikin's. While Nathan was driven by science, Ohsawa and Kushi were the products of the Oriental culture, which sees the vast patterns in the universe, and links them to personal behavior of all kinds, especially to diet. Nathan's teachings concentrated on the body, while Ohsawa and Kushi saw the union of body and spirit.

Michio Kushi began teaching the relationship between diet and health in 1949, the year he came to the United States. His was the broadest of visions. He saw the dangers of modern farming methods and supported the early organic agriculture movement in this country. He saw the need to make healthful foods available to people on a large scale and opened one of the first natural food distribution businesses, which he and his wife Aveline called Erewhon. He taught people how diet causes disease, and how it can be used to cure it. He counseled untold numbers of people with every sort of disease—many of which were termed incurable by medicine, but were later cured by following Kushi's advice.

But Michio went even further. He taught people how diet effects thinking, emotional equilibrium, and outlook on life, and how these factors effect psychological and spiritual health.

In fact, diet was only part of his teachings, albeit a major part. His central theme was the philosophy of yin and yang, the fundamental polarity of life. His goals were equally far-reaching —physical health, improved judgment, and world peace.

Kushi took these subjects to their outer limits. For literally hundreds of thousands of people, macrobiotics became part of their overall spiritual outlook; it became both compass and cure. Today, macrobiotics is the most widely practiced diet and health regimen in the world, and Michio and his wife, Aveline, continue to spread the word around the world.

There have been many other people who made the current diet and health revolution a reality. The fields of science, politics, and agriculture has seen the emergence of giants whose work has changed everything. Among them are Dr. Michael Jacobson, executive director of the Center for Science in the Public Interest. Jacobson, a microbiologist, used scientific information as it was originally intended: to improve the lot and life of our society. In politics, few people in history can claim · the kind of contribution made by George McGovern, who chaired the Senate Select Committee on Nutrition and Human Needs, and whose *Dietary Goals for the United States* created the scientific basis for the health revolution we have experienced. In agriculture, natural farmer Masanobu Fukuoka, whose *One Straw Revolution* was the seminal work in organic farming; and Robert Rodale, who pioneered the American organic farming movement, published its leading proponents (including Fukuoka), and demonstrated again and again the efficacy of organic methods.

All scientific work is important; some is more important than the rest. Dean Ornish's work ranks high on the ladder, but he stands on a ladder built by other men and women. No one exists in a vacuum, no discovery comes of itself.

But as we go forward, it is good to look around and acknowledge the work of others whose contributions have made our own lives better.

Tom Monte
Amherst, Massachusetts
January, 1991

Preface

Nearly twenty years ago, our friend Dr. William Castelli and associates at the Framingham Heart Study conducted research on members of the macrobiotic community in Boston. They tested over a hundred volunteers and were surprised to discover that their cholesterol levels were much lower than the normally high averages in the United States. Later, when Dr. Castelli visited Japan, he was met at the airport by reporters. When asked about the best way to prevent heart disease, he replied, "Just follow your traditional cuisine."

In the early 1970s, we decided to focus our macrobiotic educational programs on the connection between diet and cancer. At that time, Dr. Castelli told us that the cancer and diet relationship was somewhat complex, but that the relationship between diet and cholesterol—and by extension heart disease—was much more simple and clear. He recommended that we focus our seminars and publications on this issue. However, until now, we have not concentrated so much on the problem of cholesterol. This book, written with the help of our good friend, Tom Monte, is one of our first to discuss the relationship between diet and cholesterol in depth, and to represent the macrobiotic diet as an effective method for lowering cholesterol, promoting weight loss, and achieving natural health and beauty.

Every year, macrobiotic teachers from throughout Europe and around the world meet for the European Macrobiotic Assembly. In November, 1989, I adressed the Assembly and expressed my hope that the Berlin Wall would come down. Five days later the gate opened, and on the following year, the Assembly was held in a unified Berlin. It was a wonderful gathering at which macrobiotic teachers from Eastern Europe and the Soviet Union joined their colleagues in Western Europe. However, even with these positive developments, the world is still in a state of confusion. I decided to form a Women's Macrobiotic Society so that women around the world can speak out and communicate with each other. I believe that now is the time for women in all corners of the globe to join hands to establish health and peace throughout the world.

Forty years ago I came to this country with the dream of world health and world peace. My target was to help humanity avoid a repeat of Hiroshima and Nagasaki. I am sad that as of now, world peace still remains elusive, but at the same time I am confident that macrobiotics can help establish health and peace on the personal, family, community, and global levels in the future. As we approach to the twenty-first century, let us make our goal of the establishment of a healthy and peaceful world for future generations. It is my hope that this book can help guide us in that direction by offering a simple and practical method for achieving health, peace, and beauty in our daily lives.

Aveline Kushi
Brookline, Massachusetts
January, 1991

Acknowledgments

I am indebted for life to many friends who have made it possible for me to go on writing. I cannot acknowledge them all here, but my gratitude to them is made constant by the tremulous ground my life as a writer stands upon.

Among those I can thank here are Michio and Aveline Kushi, for their ongoing contribution to health and world peace; and Nathan and Ilene Pritikin, who will always be close to my heart. My sincere thanks and appreciation also goes to Mr. Iwao Yoshizaki and Mr. Yoshiro Fujiwara, whose publishing skills and princely patience made this book possible. Finally, my love and appreciation go to my family, who form the foundation.

Tom Monte

Contents

Chapter 10:   Cooking to Lower Cholesterol, *173*

Introduction

Many diseases states one disease

Never has there been so obvious an answer to so big a problem.

Each year, tens of millions of people die from diseases collectively called *degenerative*—illnesses such as heart disease, cancer, stroke, obesity, and adult-onset diabetes. Yet, most of these diseases are preventable and many even reversible. Of course, long before any one of these illnesses kill, they maim. They keep people from realizing their full potential. They destroy our chances at happiness.

Let us look for a moment at the most common form of degenerative disease: illnesses of the heart and arteries.

Heart disease is the greatest epidemic the human race has ever known. Almost 70 million Americans suffer from illnesses of the heart and arteries; 60 million alone suffer from high blood pressure. Each year, one million Americans die annually from illnesses of the heart and arteries, including stroke, high blood pressure, and atherosclerosis. About 1.5 million Americans annually suffer heart attacks and an estimated 500,000 of them die. In fact, cardiovascular disease accounts for one-out-of-every two deaths in the United States today. More people have been killed by diseases of the heart and arteries than all the wars in U.S. history.

Yet the cure for this terrible disease is right in front of our faces; it has been proven scientifically again and again: *Correct diet cures the most common forms of heart disease*. That is a fact. Any doctor or scientist who has examined the scientific research will tell you the same thing. Nevertheless, there are many misconceptions, great clouds of controversy, and much heated debate among people over this issue. The reason so many people are confused about the truth is because there is so much misinformation published and broadcast.

That is why we are writing this book. We want to wipe away a lot of these clouds and provide an easy-to-follow program that will help you prevent and overcome heart disease, obesity, and other serious illnesses.

The human race is in a unique period in its history. Our Western, industrialized society is like a human being who has been confronted for the first time with the overwhelming proof that his behavior for many years has been incorrect. We have all been in this situation, and it is not easy. The first time we learn that we are wrong, we rebel. We do not want to face it. We conjure up all kinds of excuses, perhaps even blame others for the mistakes we have made.

Our society is in the same situation. We are confronted with the overwhelming proof, yet many of us do not want to believe it. We rebel. Sometimes, this rebellion takes the form of misinformation: some people claim that heart disease is caused by one's genetic makeup; others say that diet cannot lower your cholesterol level enough to make a difference; others say that cholesterol level is unimportant in the treatment of heart disease. As you will see, none of this is true. But many people *want* to believe it; consequently, this false information winds up in popular magazines or newspapers or on television, and the real cure for heart disease and other illnesses is not employed by those who need it.

Heart disease, cancer, obesity, and adult-onset diabetes are all related illnesses. The causes are essentially the same. As you read this book, you will realize that *these diseases are actually one disease*.

That statement may be difficult to understand because they appear to be very different from each other. Heart disease manifests as something very different than, say, cancer. And the common cancers—cancers of the breast, colon, and prostate— seem to be unrelated. But by the time you have finished reading this book, you will see that each of these illnesses is actually a different symptom-state stemming from the same underlying disease.

That singular underlying illnesses can be called *poisoning*. We are all poisoning ourselves. As the poison increases in our bodies, it causes certain types of symptom-states: In some people, the poison causes heart disease, in others cancer; in still others, adult-onset diabetes, or high blood pressure, or stroke. The overt, or manifesting illnesses, appear quite different from each other. The symptoms appear quite different from each other. But the cause is the same: poisoning.

What is the poison we are taking in? There are several, but the most dangerous are fat and cholesterol. In very small amounts, these two food constituents are essential to health. But when we eat more fat and cholesterol than we should, they are highly toxic.

Fat and cholesterol in the diet becomes cholesterol in the blood. *The key to good health is well-nourished blood—rich in nutrients and low in cholesterol.* Fat and cholesterol are the two most damaging poisons in the diet. Therefore, we are going to concentrate on these two as the keys to good health. In addition, this book will outline a diet that can give you healthy blood.

There are other poisons that, when taken in sufficient quantities, can also be highly toxic. These include refined sugars and artificial ingredients, especially pesticides, colors, and flavors. Together, these poisons destroy life. They distort our thinking; they prevent optimal use of our talents; they weaken us physically; and they kill.

In this book, we are going to concentrate primarily on fat and cholesterol, but we will be writing about the other poisons, as well. More importantly, we are going to provide an alternative to the typical toxic diet, and an alternative to heart disease, cancer, obesity, and many other serious illnesses. That alternative is the macrobiotic diet. Our purpose is not only to say what is wrong with the current Western diet, but to describe a diet that can prevent and reverse disease.

All too often, health books tell people to eat less meat or dairy foods. They say, eat more salad, more vegetables, more bread. In other words, the diet these books recommend is virtually the same diet as most Americans are already eating. The only difference is that it contains less of certain foods. Consequently, tens of thousands of people today are eating at the periphery of the standard Western diet—they are eating more salads, more packaged vegetables, more bread and potatoes, and smaller amounts of red meat, eggs, dairy products, and sugar. At the same time, they expect this diet to do them some good. But it does not work. People do not experience any real improvement of their health, energy levels, and weight. More importantly, they get tired of eating salads and potatoes. Pretty soon, they cannot stand it. They give up the whole effort; they throw up their hands and yell, "It's impossible to eat right."

The problem is this: you cannot sustain a diet that is filled with "don'ts"—do not eat this food or that one. It is sort of like being invited to a banquet and not being allowed to eat anything but the salad.

The macrobiotic diet is much easier to follow because it is a complete break with the typical American regimen. Moreover, it is filled with "dos"—*do* eat whole grains, vegetables, beans, sea vegetables, fruit, natural condiments, natural sweeteners, and fish. The sheer variety of the macrobiotic diet is remarkable. Once you become acquainted with the vegetable kingdom, and adept at preparing such foods, you will marvel at the variety of tastes and textures available in such a diet.

Another problem with diets is that they are geared toward dealing with only one type of problem. For example, some people are interested only in losing weight. So they sign up with one of the weight reducing programs that recommend diets high in protein and low in carbohydrates. They eat lots of meat, eggs, and dairy, and less bread, potatoes, and grains. These diets say that protein causes weight loss, while carbohydrate-rich foods cause weight gain. People who adopt these diets do in fact lose weight for awhile, but the weight loss is temporary—it consists almost exclusively of water retention—and as we will see throughout this book, the damage such foods do to health is extensive.

The macrobiotic diet is a healing diet. It is also a diet you can stay on for the rest of your life. Once you fully adopt the macrobiotic diet, you can stop worrying about your cholesterol level, your weight, and a lot of other health concerns. You can eat until you are satisfied and still lose weight, lower your cholesterol, and reduce your risk of contracting any number of degenerative diseases, including cancer. The macrobiotic diet is delicious, satisfying, and easy to follow. The only drawback to it is that it requires you to establish a whole new set of habits. That requires a certain amount of time to adjust to a new set of flavors and foods. But food preferences are not genetically controlled. They are learned. As long as you give yourself a chance to gradually adapt to your new macrobiotic diet, you will wonder how you ever ate any other way. You will find the food delicious, fully satisfying, and health enhancing.

Once you have established these new habits, macrobiotics is as easy to prepare and follow as your current diet is. And the rewards are life changing.

As you will notice, our book is divided into ten chapters. Each chapter is organized in a simple question and answer format. We begin with the most simple questions and work up to the more complex ones. You will understand the cause of serious illnesses, the macrobiotic approach to these problems, and the scientific evidence supporting that approach.

Chapters 8, 9, and 10 describe the diet and menus in detail. It offers a detailed program that includes menu plans and easy-to-follow recipes. The menu plans provide for ten days of three meals per day. We recommend that you follow these menu plans for 30 days. If you follow this program for 30 days, you will begin to see real proof of how effective macrobiotics is at changing your life. Give the macrobiotic diet one month—just 30 days—and it will change your life for the better.

So, let us begin. Let us turn the page and start a new life.

Chapter 1

To Go Where the Blood Goes: A Cautionary Tale of Oxygen, Cells, Arteries, and Cholesterol

Human life requires oxygen. Of all the things that we need for our survival—including food, clothing, and shelter—our demand for oxygen is the most immediate. We need oxygen in vast quantities and we need it now—not ten minutes from now. Generally, when we think of our need for oxygen, we think of breathing and we think of our lungs. We do not think of our cells. But our cells are the reason we breathe. Oxygen is drawn into the lungs and taken up by the blood, which in turn transports the oxygen to several-trillion cells that make up the human body.

There are many ways of understanding health and illness. One way is to simply ask yourself how you feel. Another way is to understand what is happening in your blood and your cells. Ironically, these two may contradict each other. The reason is that while you may feel good today, there may be things occurring in your cells that will make you feel ill tomorrow. One of the most important factors that affects your blood and cells is your daily food. To a large extent, our diets control our ability to prevent and even reverse disease.

To better understand what our food is doing to us, let us take an imaginary journey. Let us go where the oxygen goes and see what takes place inside the body.

Imagine that you can shrink yourself and a submarine to microscopic size. Now imagine further that you are inside this microscopic submarine, which is then swallowed by another human being, a young man of about twenty-five years of age. Our friend is relatively healthy, though slightly overweight. He works in an office and outside the normal chores of home and work, he is not particularly active.

The headlights on your tiny submarine illuminate your incredible journey through the esophagus, the stomach, and into the small intestine, where you and your submarine are absorbed into the person's bloodstream. Suddenly, you find yourself traveling inside a dynamic red liquid, filled with disk-like red blood cells—huge saucers that fly by. There are also a variety of great lumbering white cells that patrol the blood looking for foreign invaders—including tiny submarines, such as ours! Fortunately, we are protected by the power of the imagination. There are also myriad other entities, such as dead or broken cells, vitamins and minerals, squiggly, snake-like proteins, and blood platelets, called *thrombocytes*—all of them floating in this red ocean world. This is a marvelous universe, so rich and complex, so filled with myriad forms of life.

You decide to dock onto a red blood cell. You witness its donut shape and its red luminous pigment, in which iron and oxygen are carried. The blood rushes along on its long journey through the universe of the human body.

Suddenly, there is a bend in the blood vessel. The vessel narrows considerably and then heads toward a tiny opening, perhaps half the size of your red blood cell. It seems too small for your red blood cell to pass through. You realize that this small passageway is the opening to a capillary, a tiny vessel that allows blood and oxygen to nourish a specific set of cells. You quickly calculate the size of a red blood cell: 7.5 microns in diameter. Then you calculate the size of a capillary: 3.5 microns in diameter. Uh, oh. Will our red blood cell make it, or will there be a sudden crash? You brace yourself for the impact as the cell races toward the tiny opening. Suddenly, with almost miraculous dexterity, your red blood cell folds in half. It squeezes into the little vessel. You are snug inside the capillary, but still moving. Now your red cell is rubbing up against the capillary wall, a semi-permeable membrane through which oxygen can pass from red blood cells to body cells, also called somatic cells.

As your red cell brushes up against one of the cells, it gives up its supply of oxygen to the cell. In return, the cell gives its supply of carbon dioxide to the red blood cell. You witness this awesome exchange and experience firsthand the somatic cell's gasping for life as it gratefully absorbs the oxygen from the red cell. Meanwhile, other red cells make the same exchange to neighboring somatic cells. Immediately, each somatic cell is revived and enlivened by the intake of oxygen. You marvel at the coordination of this exchange: oxygen—life!—in exchange for carbon dioxide. All the cells are being provided for by the blood. Each cell is accounted for, each receives its supply of life-giving oxygen. There is something wonderful about the process; implicit in this remarkable event is a certain joy.

Once the exchange of oxygen for carbon dioxide is made, you notice a change in the red cell. It goes from being bright red to a dark, almost purplish color. The carbon dioxide has changed the color of the blood! It now contains the burden of the cell's waste. Your red cell immediately hurries onward, toward the lungs, where it will be able to give up its carbon dioxide load, and be infused with another quantity of oxygen, which will start the cycle again.

Your red cell makes its way out of the capillary and into a larger vessel and then to an artery where its speed increases dramatically. Woosh! Woosh! Every heartbeat sends a rush of energy through the bloodstream, driving the plasma and cells onward in great and powerful waves.

Finally, you reach the heart. There are four chambers of the heart. You enter the heart by flowing into the right atrium chamber. Suddenly, the atrium contracts, pushing the blood past the tricuspid valve and into the right ventricle chamber. Now the pulmonary valve opens, and you rush into the pulmonary artery and on to the lungs. There you pass through the seemingly endless maze of the lung's alveoli, where you witness another incredible exchange—this one is the opposite of the one before: red blood cells are giving up their carbon dioxide load for oxygen. The red blood cell you are riding pulls up into an alleyway—a tiny alveoli where it surrenders its carbon dioxide and receives a fresh infusion of oxygen. Once again, your red cell is clean, bright red, and rich with vitality. You sense its restored energy as it hurries out of the lungs and back to the heart.

You enter into the left atrium, the atrium contracts, and you are pushed passed the mitral valve and into the left ventricle. Now the left ventricle contracts and you ride the wave of blood passed the aortic valve and into the aorta. This is a big super-highway. You explode onto the superhighway and, once again, you are on your way to the cells of the body, along the body's circulatory canals.

The blood is on a mission! You make your way from the big superhighways, the arteries, to the smaller country roads, the vessels, and finally to the back alleys of the human body again: the capillaries.

As your red blood cell approaches a capillary, you notice something odd taking place. There is a bottleneck of some kind. A huge congestion is occurring right before the tiny entrance to the capillary. There is an incredible traffic jam and you are being drawn into it. Everything is stuck! A great number of disk-like red blood cells have all been stuck together. They are all flattened against each other. They look like a huge roll of coins, each one pressed flat against the other. As such, they are incapable of bending and fitting into the tiny capillary. Instead, this roll of cells resembles an enormous bus stuck before a tiny bicycle path. It cannot go forward. Meanwhile, the press of traffic from behind prevents it from going backward. Every-thing is bottled up. If blood does not get inside that capillary, cells may suffocate and die.

What has caused this mess? Why have all these red blood cells clumped together like this?

Suddenly, you realize that there is something very sticky in the blood itself—tiny balls of fat, called chylomicrons, are raining down upon the red blood cells and causing them to stick together like glue. The chylomicrons are coming down like snow. This moist glue is causing other cells to stick to each other, too. It is a mess. The cells are glued together into one large clump at the bottleneck of this capillary.

All at once, you realize what has happened. Our friend—whose body you are traveling in—has been eating cheese! Or drinking a glass of milk! Or eating a steak! Eeee gads! The fat from one or more of these foods has passed into the bloodstream and is causing havoc. Fat and cholesterol are gunking up the works!

You decide to turn on your engines and let go of your red blood cell, which is immobilized by the congestion, and pass along with the plasma. You make your way to the opening of the tiny capillary and squeeze past the red blood cells so that you can enter the little vessel. What you see now is horrible. The cells that await oxygen and nutrition are all suffocating. They are dark with the poison of carbon dioxide. They gasp for any trace of oxygen in the blood, but there is none. The red blood cells, which would bring the oxygen, are all stuck at the entrance way to the capillary. They are all blocked. Consequently, no oxygen can get in to these cells. Now the cells inside are dying, each one suffocating in a slow, painful death. One by one, they expire. Whole groups of cells die. You gun your engines and get away from this terrible scene.

Once away from the mass execution of cells, you realize that you have just witnessed the "rouleaux" effect—the bottlenecking of red blood cells, caused by the consumption of a single fatty food or meal. Rouleaux, a French word for roll, or roll of coins, is used to describe the adherence of red cells that are stuck together by the tiny balls of fat that infuse the blood after a meal rich in fat or cholesterol. The result is the dramatic diminution of oxygen to cells, causing some cells to die of suffocation.

You speed up your submarine and leave this land of the dead for better parts.

On your way, you see other cells suffocating for breath. At one such place, you notice a strange sight: deformed cells. These cells that are getting just enough oxygen to survive, but they are growing in strange ways, and in very disorderly patterns, so different from the beautiful mosaics that cells normally form. The deformed cells grow in bunches, cramming each other for space. They are competing with each other for the available nutrients, fighting for oxygen and life. Meanwhile, a host of immune cells—macrophage cells, B cells that make antibodies, and killer Ts that destroy pathogens and aberrant cells—are mobilized against these deformed cells, attacking them.

A war is going on right before your eyes, and that war is cancer. A few cells have become aberrant, their DNA deformed from lack of oxygen and other hostile conditions within their environment. They have grown disorganized and mutant ways and must be stopped. The alternative is the death of the entire organism. The white blood cells will likely win this battle. The cancer cells will be eliminated soon. But what about the next time, or a few years from now?

You decide to take a trip north, to the heart, and soon find yourself inside one of the three main coronary arteries that provide blood, oxygen, and nutrients to the heart muscle. Once inside the long artery you recognize the topography is highly irregular. You have noticed this in other arteries, too, but here the irregularity is worse: tall yellow mountains growing up out of the walls of the artery. You realize gloomily that these yellow mountains are atherosclerosis: cholesterol plaque that is growing inside this young man's arteries.

If this young man continues to eat a high fat diet, these yellow mountains will continue to grow. At some point, part of the mountainous boil may break off, float further down the artery, and block the flow of blood to the heart, causing a heart attack. Or another scenario is possible: the boils can become so large that they cut off the flow of blood to the heart or brain entirely, causing a part of the heart or brain to die from lack of oxygen; in other words, a heart attack or stroke.

We already know that our friend is overweight. Consequently, we know that his heart is laboring under the burden of excess fat surrounding the heart and making it even more difficult to pump blood. The heart is already troubled by the diminished quantity of oxygen resulting from the atherosclerosis in the coronary arteries.

You leave the heart area and take an artery and a few veins to the periphery of the body and see the adipose tissue, the tissues where fat is stored in large cells. These cells are huge—great bags of yellow fat. Inside these fat cells are all sorts of objects, such as carbon and radioactive particles. There is also pools of chemicals: you notice pesticides, such as DDT, and lots of industrial waste, including PCBs (polychlorinated biphenyls—a powerful carcinogen). This is a garbage dump! The body's waste station.

Suddenly, you come upon a radioactive element that is emitting radiation. Electrons are flying by you like bullets. They strike other fat cells. Some strike the nucleus of a cell and kill it instantly. Others strike the cell and cause it to become deformed. Radioactivity is one of the most powerful carcinogens known to mankind. This is how it causes cells to mutate: by striking the nucleus and causing aberrant cell division.

As you tour these hideous masses of fat, you realize that contained in all this fat is every kind of pollutant our friend has come in contact with since he was a child. It is all stored here, thanks in a large part to all the fat in his diet and his overweight condition. Fat traps these pollutants and holds them in its grip, until the day that it releases some highly toxic material into the bloodstream where it lodges elsewhere in the body and causes an illness, such as cancer. Unless he eliminates these toxins safely through the intestinal tract, these pollutants may cause some serious illness later. In other words, our friend may be a walking time bomb.

Through the magic of your imagination, you manage to shrink yourself and your submarine still further. You are now so small that you can see the world of molecules. This is the world of spheres. It is like traveling in space between planets. In fact, most of what you see now is open space. Distances are marked by great atomic spheres—electrons that, like moons, orbit atomic nuclei, each made up of protons and neutrons, which resemble a cluster of planets. The electrons are moving so rapidly that one dare not get near its path. Your submarine is now a spaceship and you marvel at the tremendous energy of this world, generated of course by the movement of these atomic particles. Each sphere spins like an endless set of gyroscopes, perfectly balanced. It is a world of such brilliant color and light that your mind boggles.

As you travel in this world of orbiting lights, you approach a great disturbance. Electrons are being released from their natural orbit. An atom is literally decaying. The electrons are firing off chaotically in all directions.

Atoms must have the same number of electrons (or negatively charged particles) as they do protons (or positively charged particles). The loss of each electron creates an imbalance in the atom. In order to restore balance, the atom must find another electron to replace the missing electron. To do this, atoms are attaching themselves to other nearby atoms, creating chemical bonds that did not exist before. More electrons are released, more instability takes place. Some atoms are stealing electrons from neighboring atoms to restore their own balance. There is utter chaos. It is a riot of atomic activity. The new chemical bonds can reshape DNA and cause cell mutations. One such mutation is cancer.

You realize that this atomic chaos that you are looking at is free radical formation. These electrons, called free radicals, are being released because each fat molecule is becoming rancid. It is literally decaying inside this person's flesh. You remember the research being done at the University of California at Los Angeles (UCLA) and other major universities (about which, more later), where scientists are saying that more than 60 illnesses—including heart disease and cancer—are caused by free radical formation. Immediately, you understand the process. Electrons, suddenly freed from their orbits, strike other cells, sometimes disturbing DNA, which in turn causes uncontrolled cell growth and malignancy.

This free radical formation is taking place throughout the body, in the intestines, in the lungs, in the sexual organs—everywhere that excess fat accumulates and decays.

This young man is killing himself and he does not even know it. But long before he dies, he will gradually weaken unnecessarily. If he continues to eat the food he so enjoys—fatty fast foods, eggs, bacon, steaks, and other animal foods—he will slowly decline over many years, losing strength, mental alertness, and much of his youthful vitality. His mind will become more dull; his body less responsive; his sexual vitality will weaken and perhaps wane entirely (healthy circulation is essential to male sexual vitality); he will carry around pounds of unnecessary fat, while the cholesterol plaques in his veins and arteries prevent blood from flowing to the heart, brain, and other vital organs throughout the body. It will be a fast aging and a slow death.

By his own hand—or rather, his own hand and mouth.

The irony is that all of this is that the degeneration process can be halted and disease can be prevented. Serious illnesses can even be reversed. Health can be restored. But for that to happen, our friend must change his ways—before it is too late.

Chapter 2

All about Fat, Cholesterol, and Cardiovascular Disease

The food we eat and the activities we perform determine the quantity of oxygen that gets to our cells, including our heart. As we will see later on, even the thoughts we think effect the quantity of oxygen that flows to our cells.

The food constituents that most effect oxygen and blood flow are fat and cholesterol, but heart disease is only one of the many illnesses that can result from the overconsumption of fat and cholesterol.

Let us begin by looking carefully at fat and cholesterol and see how they influence the health of our heart. In later chapters, we look at how foods rich in fat and cholesterol give rise to other diseases, including cancer, diabetes, obesity, and some of the illnesses associated with aging, such as arthritis, hearing and sight loss, and senility.

In this chapter, we are going to start by asking some basic questions and then answering them, beginning with the simplest of all:

What is cholesterol?

Cholesterol is a yellowish, wax-like substance that your body uses to create hormones, bile acids, and cell membranes.

Much of the cholesterol in your blood is actually produced by your liver, but all cells produce some cholesterol. In addition, you get even more cholesterol from many of the foods you eat.

Doctors and scientists often refer to cholesterol as dietary cholesterol, which comes from food, or serum cholesterol, which is the cholesterol in your blood.

What is LDL cholesterol and HDL cholesterol?

Cholesterol is often differentiated as LDL, meaning, low density lipoprotein, and HDL, which stands for high density lipoprotein.

Actually, neither LDL nor HDL is cholesterol, but proteins that carry cholesterol to specific places. LDL carries cholesterol to your vessels and arteries, while HDL carries cholesterol out of your body. LDL gives rise to the disease called atherosclerosis, or cholesterol plaques that clog the arteries throughout the body, especially the arteries that bring blood to the heart. These plaques are like boils that grow inside the walls of the arteries. Eventually, they can grow so large that they can block blood flow to tissues and organs, such as the heart and brain. When blood flow to the heart or brain is blocked, the person usually experiences a heart attack or stroke, respectively. (We will talk more about atherosclerosis and how it manifests later in this chapter.)

LDL is often referred to as the "bad cholesterol" because leads to atherosclerosis, the underlying illness for most heart disease.

HDL is often called "good cholesterol" because it brings cholesterol to the intestinal tract, where it is eliminated through the feces. In this way, HDL lowers the amount of cholesterol in your bloodstream.

LDL cholesterol increases when we eat foods rich in saturated fat and cholesterol. HDL increases as a result of exercise. (We will talk more about exercise in a later chapter.) Consequently, the more you exercise, the greater your HDL levels, which increases your ability to eliminate cholesterol from your body.

Some studies have shown that moderate alcohol consumption decreases the incidence of heart disease, while other studies have shown no positive effects from alcohol, and some have demonstrated a negative effect of alcohol, even for moderate imbibers. Some scientists have said that alcohol has a positive effect on the heart because it raises HDLs.

There is no question that regular consumption of alcohol has an adverse effect on the heart, as well as many other organs, including kidneys and sexual organs. (In men, alcohol shrinks testicles and adversely effects hormones. Alcohol stops the pituitary gland from stimulating the testes to create testosterone.)

Alcohol causes blood vessels to harden and the body to retain water, causing increased strain on the kidneys and heart.

Alcohol does raise HDLs, but not the type that effects your overall blood cholesterol level. There are a variety of HDLs, some of which have little or no effect on overall blood cholesterol. Alcohol tends to raise these high density lipoproteins. Consequently, alcohol has little positive effect on blood cholesterol.

Nevertheless, even the good HDLs will not be of much benefit if you continue to eat a high fat and high cholesterol diet.

The reason is that exercise will not lower your overall LDL cholesterol level enough to make a difference in your health. HDL will only enhance your ability to eliminate cholesterol from your body. If you eat a high fat diet, your LDL cholesterol will remain high enough to overwhelm the good that HDL is doing you. This is why so many long distance runners with high LDL and HDL cholesterol levels have heart attacks. Despite their HDLs, they still suffer from atherosclerosis, which blocks blood flow to the heart. Remember, that cholesterol is not burned as fuel. You do not actually reduce your cholesterol level from exercise. Only dietary change or cholesterol-lowering drugs can lower your cholesterol level. But cholesterol-lowering drugs have severe side effects, while diet is every bit as effective at lowering cholesterol, yet has only positive side effects. Exercise is important for other reasons, too, which we will discuss in the chapter on exercise. Still, it is important to keep in mind that exercise will not save you from heart disease, no matter how much you exercise.

The best examples of this are long distance runner Jim Fixx, author of *The Complete Book of Running* (Random House, 1977), and tennis great Arthur Ashe. Both men had reached the very pinnacle of their sports. Their physical conditioning had reached Herculean heights—except for their hearts. Both men ate extremely high fat diets. In an interview with the *London Daily*

Mail in 1979, Jim Fixx told a reporter that he ate eggs, bacon, sausage, buttered toast, and coffee with cream for breakfast and that he enjoyed high fat meals all the time. "If you run, you can participate fully in the ways of our civilization and get away with it," he told the reporter.

In July 1984, Jim Fixx died of a massive heart attack at the age of 52. His cholesterol level at the time of his death was 253 mg/dl, a level that cardiologists state is eight times as likely to cause a heart attack than 160 mg/dl. Just before his death, Fixx was warned to change his diet and lower his cholesterol level, but he pooh-poohed this advice, saying that those who urged runners to alter their eating habits were just trying to scare people.

Arthur Ashe was only 36 when he suffered a massive heart attack. One of the three main arteries leading to his heart was completely closed off by atherosclerosis, a consequence of his high fat diet, and brought on his heart attack. Ashe underwent bypass surgery. Fortunately, he survived the heart attack and the surgery and has since changed his way of eating. He has publically encouraged others to do the same.

When you exercise, your heart works harder and consequently its need for oxygen increases. If one or more of the arteries leading to the heart are blocked, less blood will flow to the heart, and the muscle will not get sufficient oxygen to nourish the muscle. This can cause a heart attack.

Why does the heart need oxygen?

All cells need oxygen to burn carbohydrates for fuel. The heart is no different in this regard. But the heart also needs oxygen to support its role as an electrical pump. Oxygen ions are used to maintain the electrical charge necessary to keep the pump working. This electrical charge fires along a kind of fibrous wiring within the heart muscle, and makes the heart's contraction and expansion—its beating—possible.

Three main arteries, called coronary arteries, provide blood and oxygen flow to the heart. As long as blood flows equally through these three arteries, the heart muscle gets equal amounts of oxygen to all its parts. This makes coordinated, or rhythmic beating possible. Even if the blood does not flow evenly, the heart will still work adequately, *as long as you do not overwork the heart.*

During exercise, the heart muscle requires more oxygen to support its increased beating.

If, due to atherosclerosis, one of the arteries to the heart is 90 percent closed, while another is 40 percent closed, this will ensure differing amounts of oxygen to the heart muscle. Part of the heart will get far less oxygen than another part. Consequently, the electrical charge becomes imbalanced and uncoordinated and one part of the heart beats at a different rate than another. As the uncoordinated condition persists, the heart may skip a beat. This abnormal rhythm is called *arrhythmia.*

Arrhythmia is one of the most common causes of heart attack. It accounts for more than 400,000 sudden deaths each year.

Uncoordinated beating can also take place when one of the arteries is closed off entirely, thus preventing blood and oxygen from flowing to the heart at all. This will suffocate and kill one part of the heart, and also bring on a heart attack.

All of this is caused by atherosclerosis, or cholesterol plaques forming within the coronary arteries. And atherosclerosis is caused by too much cholesterol in the bloodstream.

What determines the quantity of cholesterol in my blood?

Both fat and cholesterol in food are converted by the body into blood cholesterol. All animal foods—red meat, dairy products, eggs, chicken, and fish—contain cholesterol. There is no cholesterol in vegetable foods—grains, beans, vegetables, or fruits.

However, all foods—including vegetable foods—contain varying amounts of fat. In general, animal foods are rich in fat, except for fish. Most fish are low to moderate in fat content.

On the other hand, most of the vegetable-kingdom foods —whole grains, beans, vegetables, and fruits—are very low in fat. Consequently, people who consume only vegetable foods usually have very low cholesterol levels. People who eat vegetable foods and fish also have very low cholesterol levels.

Certain vegetable foods, however, are high in fat. All nuts and seeds contain moderate to high levels of fat. Coconut, avocadoes, and olives are rich in fat. And some vegetable oils contain a specific kind of fat that you want to avoid—saturated fat. These include coconut oil, palm oil, and palm kernel oil.

What is the difference between fats, such as saturated and polyunsaturated?

When it comes to fat, you must be concerned with two things: the quantity and type.

There are three kinds of fats—polyunsaturated, found mostly in vegetables; monounsaturated, found mostly in oils; and saturated fats, found mostly in animal foods and in coconut oil, palm oil, and palm kernel oil. Apart from these oils, vegetables do not contain saturated fat.

Chemically, saturated fats are different from unsaturated fats in that their string of carbon and oxygen atoms are filled to capacity, or saturated, with hydrogen atoms. This makes the saturated fat more dense than unsaturated fats and, consequently, causes it to remain a solid at room temperature.

Saturated fats dramatically raise blood cholesterol levels and are the most dangerous food substance there is. (As we will see, excess consumption of saturated fat causes heart disease, cancer, high blood pressure, diabetes, arthritis, immune deficiencies, and obesity.) Saturated fat is not fully broken down by the body and consequently it cannot be digested. Much of the fat we eat is not eliminated from the body, but instead makes its way into the bloodstream as tiny microns of fat, called *chylomicrons*. These chylomicrons adhere to the red blood cells and the walls of vessels, where they form atherosclerotic plaque.

Saturated fat also collects along the walls of the intestines, lining the intestinal cells with a layer of fat, which prevents efficient absorption of nutrients from food.

For these reasons and many more, we must be careful with

all red meat, dairy products, eggs, and chicken, all of which contain saturated fat.

Most fish, on the other hand, are lean and much of the fat is polyunsaturated. But there is some saturated fat, especially in the meatier fish, such as mackerel and herring.

Polyunsaturated fats have the fewest hydrogen atoms within the molecular structure and are therefore the least dense of fats. Polyunsaturated fats are found in vegetable foods and cold water fish, such as cod, flounder, salmon, haddock, and scrod. The white-meat fish, such as cod, haddock, flounder, scrod, trout, and perch are low in all fats.

Polyunsaturated fats lower blood cholesterol levels. That means that all vegetable foods and many fish will lower your cholesterol level. Salmon, for example, contains an oil called *omega-3 polyunsaturated fat*, which has been shown to lower cholesterol levels.

Still, all fats should be held to a minimum. Excess consumption of polyunsaturated fats has been linked to cancer. (See section on cancer in Chapter 5.) Polyunsaturated fats also cause sludging of the red blood cells—the rouleaux effect (explained in Chapter 1 and in greater detail below). Only small amounts of polyunsaturated or vegetable fats are recommended. (See dietary guidelines described in Chapter 8.)

In general, the body handles polyunsaturated fats much more efficiently when the rest of the diet is low in saturated fat. If there is a lot of saturated fat in the diet, the polyunsaturated fat becomes more dangerous.

Monounsaturated fats, which are found primarily in oils, such as olive, rapeseed (canola), sunflower, and safflower oils, have more hydrogen atoms in their molecule and are thus more viscous than polyunsaturated oils. Monounsaturated fats have no effect on blood cholesterol.

All oils are fats, except that oil is liquid at room temperature, while fat is solid. Sometimes you will see on a food label the words "partially hydrogenated" oils. This means that the fat contained in this food has been saturated with more hydrogen atoms, which has made the food more dense or solid at room temperature. Margarines are often hydrogenated, so that they will be thicker and behave more like butter, a food that has a great deal of saturated fat. When an oil has been hydrogenated, it is more saturated, and hence more unhealthful.

All saturated fats and cholesterol will raise your blood cholesterol. The more saturated fat- and cholesterol-rich foods you eat, the higher your blood cholesterol level will be.

Which food is worse for you: saturated fat or cholesterol?

Both foods will raise blood cholesterol, but since there is more saturated fat than cholesterol in most animal foods, saturated fat is what we should be most concerned about. (The only exception to this is organ meats, brains, and kidneys, which are loaded with cholesterol.)

I thought that cholesterol level was controlled by my genes. Is that not so?

Many people believe that blood cholesterol is controlled entirely by our genes; these people also believe that diet has little or nothing to do with it. That is false. There is a genetic component to cholesterol control; the body does, after all, produce its own cholesterol. It is directed to do this by its genes. However, in most of us, that constituents a limited portion of the cholesterol that is in our blood. The rest of the cholesterol in our bodies arrives there via our diets.

Many people with high cholesterol levels say that they have genetically controlled cholesterol levels. "I can't get my cholesterol down," they say, "because my genes cause my body to produce too much cholesterol. A low fat and low cholesterol diet won't work for me."

That is also false for the vast majority of us, even the vast majority of us who have very high cholesterol levels.

According to the National Heart, Lung and Blood Institute (NHLBI), only about one-in-every-five-hundred people have familial hypercholesteremia, or genetically high cholesterol levels.

The rest of us, which makes up more than 99 percent of the population, have cholesterol levels that are controlled to a greater extent by our diets.

Those people who suffer from familial hypercholesteremia—or genetically high cholesterol—have cholesterol levels that exceed 300 mg/dl. But do not jump to conclusions if your cholesterol level is that high or higher. NHLBI scientists are quick to point out that not everyone with a cholesterol level of 300 or more has familial hypercholesteremia. In fact, only a small fraction of the people with this dangerously high cholesterol level suffer from familial hypercholesteremia. Consequently, the chances of you being one of them is exceedingly small.

Obviously, you should consult your physician if your cholesterol level is over 220 mg/dl, and especially if it is over 260 mg/dl. However, a low fat and low cholesterol diet is a necessity even for the small percentage of people with genetically high cholesterol levels. If their bodies are producing too much cholesterol as it is, such people do not need any more cholesterol from their diets.

Besides fatty foods and foods rich in cholesterol, what other foods effect my blood cholesterol level?

Decaffeinated coffee and sugar are two foods that raise blood cholesterol levels, yet have no fat.

Refined sugars also raise blood cholesterol slightly. The body converts refined sugars into triglycerides, or fatty acids. A percentage of these fatty acids—usually about 20 percent—are converted into blood cholesterol. Excess consumption of refined white sugar and fruit sugars will flood the blood with triglycerides which in turn will raise blood cholesterol somewhat. Sugar does not raise blood cholesterol to the extent that fat and cholesterol does. However, sugar has many deleterious effects, as we show later on.

Studies have shown that decaffeinated coffee raises blood cholesterol significantly.

Foods rich in protein—such as all red meat, eggs, chicken,

and dairy products—create fat. Protein is used by the body for cell replacement and repair. If you eat more protein than you need, your body will take the excess protein and convert it to fat. The fat in your tissues can raise your blood cholesterol. (See Chapter 5 for a fuller discussion of protein and the nutrient content of foods.)

What is fat used for by the body?

Our bodies use fat as a reserve fuel, a spare tank so to speak. The body's primary fuel, the one it prefers above all others, is carbohydrates, found in whole grains, beans, vegetables, and fruits. The reason carbohydrates are preferred is that they provide lots of energy and only two by-products, water and carbon dioxide, both of which the body easily eliminates.

When our carbohydrate supply has been exhausted, the body begins to burn stored energy in the form of fat. This is why exercise causes people to lose weight; because exercise causes us to burn off our carbohydrate-energy supply first, and then expend our fuel reserves, which are fat.

The body also uses fat to metabolize vitamins A, D, E, and K.

The question is: How much fat and cholesterol do we need?

Let us dispense with the easy part of that question first. The body will produce all the cholesterol it needs. There is no health reason to eat cholesterol-rich foods, such as eggs, beef, chicken, or dairy products. Since all foods contain some fat, the body will produce all the cholesterol it needs from the grains and vegetables you eat. Consequently, you do not have to worry about getting too little cholesterol. It cannot be done. But as a rule of thumb, you should not eat any more than 100 milligrams of cholesterol per day. That is a lot of cholesterol, actually. You would have to eat a small piece of fish—about three to four ounces—each day to get that much cholesterol.

It is wiser to limit animal foods to once or twice a week. This ensures that you are getting only the smallest amounts of fat and cholesterol in your diet, and that your blood cholesterol will be low. (The average American gets anywhere from 300 to 600 milligrams of cholesterol per day. That almost guarantees illness.)

How much fat do we need?

Fat is essential to human health, but we only need very small amounts of it. Since all foods contain some fat, it is virtually impossible to be depleted in fat. When we examine the eating habits around the world, we do not see any illnesses related to too little fat. Some South American tribes, for example, have existed on as little as 3 to 5 percent of their total calorie intake coming from fat, which means that the vast majority of their diets came from vegetables, fruits, and grains.

Throughout history, the human race has existed on very little fat—anywhere from 10 to 20 percent of their total calories.

Up until the twentieth century, the vast majority of people ate mostly vegetable foods, and the central food for all people was grain. In addition to grain, the human race has always depended upon vegetables—leafy greens, carrots, and potatoes, for example—and beans, and fruits as the remaining sources of nutrition.

Why this dependence upon grain? you might ask.

The answer is simple enough: Agriculture literally made civilization possible. Before men and women cultivated the earth, they were hunter-gatherers, eating wild plants and animals. They followed the herds and the seasons. They had no home. But 6,000 years ago, in Mesopotamia, where the Tigris and Euphrates rivers run, mankind learned to grow wheat. That changed everything. Grain literally gave man a home. It made him stay put. He farmed the land, learned about the seasons, the weather cycles, the plants, and their seeds. Mankind came to understand nature. This was an awesome step in consciousness. The cultivation of grain awakened men and women to their link with nature.

Grains, vegetables, and fruits were renewable foods—they could be cultivated in abundance, year after year. They could also be stored during winter.

Animals, on the other hand, were not so easily obtained, and therefore far more expensive. If you owned a pig or a cow or an ox, you were careful with how you used it. An ox could be used to help pull a cart or a plow; a pig could be sold or bartered. In other words, livestock represented wealth. People did not slaughter their animals so that they could eat steak or hamburgers every day. Only the rich could afford to eat meat on a regular basis. The peasants went weeks and even months without tasting meat, and when they did it was usually cut into small bits and cooked in soup or as part of porridge. (Even in modern times, people living in poor countries rarely eat meat. Meat is the food of affluence—just ask any Russian.)

In traditional times, people relied upon grains and vegetables as their daily foods. Animal foods were consumed as part of a celebration. Then the people slaughtered an animal and prepared the food with such care that the cooking alone reached ceremonial proportions. (One need only read the Bible or other traditional religious texts to understand how pre-modern people used animal foods in feasting, and grain in sacred rituals. Virtually all the religious ceremonies of the world involve grain: unleavened bread, or *mana* is used among Jews; consecrated bread among Christians; rice as the sacrifice to the ancestors among Orientals—these are but a few of the common uses of grain in religious ceremonies, which demonstrate the attitude of pre-modern people toward this food.)

The earth provided grain and vegetables in abundance, and therefore these foods formed the center of all traditional diets. In the East, the grains were rice and wheat; in Europe, they were wheat, oats, barley, and rye; in Africa, millet and sorghum; in the Americas, corn, and later wheat, rice, oats, and barley.

One animal food was eaten in abundance, and that was fish. For people who lived near the ocean, near lakes, and rivers, fish comprised a central part of the diet. Fish is very low in fat, however. Most fish derive less than 20 percent of their calories from fat, and usually that fat is polyunsaturated fat, which tends to lower cholesterol level.

Because the diets of people throughout most of our history

has been composed chiefly of vegetable foods and fish, the blood cholesterol level of humans throughout evolution has been exceedingly low.

Even today, we can see how low by examining the blood samples of traditional peoples of the East, South America, and certain African tribes. Among these peoples, blood cholesterol rarely gets above 140 milligrams per deciliter of blood. The average Americans blood cholesterol is about 212 milligrams per deciliter of blood.

Consequently, traditional people experience extremely low rates of heart disease, cancer, arthritis, high blood pressure, and obesity. In fact, these illnesses are largely unheard of among peoples whose diets are made up principally of whole grains, vegetables, fruits, and fish.

How much fat and cholesterol is too much for my health?

During the past fifty years, modern agriculture has managed to produce animal foods in unprecedented abundance. This remarkable feat has made it possible for people to eat red meat, eggs, chicken, and dairy products as easily as people ate grain or vegetables in previous times. In fact, people can now eat red meat three times a day, and many people do. But animal foods are extremely high in fat and cholesterol, consequently, their effects on blood cholesterol is to drive it upward.

Daily consumption of any animal foods—including red meat, eggs, and dairy products—is unhealthful.

As we said, our recommendation (see suggested dietary guidelines) is that animal foods should be included in the diet no more than twice a week.

Let us see why.

To understand how much fat is in a food, scientists often compare the calories coming from the fat of that food, to the total calories in the food itself. A food that is low in fat will have less than 20 percent of its calories coming from fat. The rest of the calories will come from other sources, such as carbohydrates or protein. A food that has a lot of fat will have 30 percent or more of its calories in fat.

Your average steak has anywhere from 40 to 70 percent of its total calories in fat, which means nearly half or more of the steak's calories go into your body in the form of fat.

Fat is also measured in grams per serving. One ounce equals about 28 grams (28.35 ounces, to be exact). At first glance, a gram seems pretty small, but when you consider that you can get several ounces of fat in one fast food meal, you begin to realize that those grams add up pretty quickly.

As a rule, animal foods are loaded with fat.

For example, stewing beef derives as much as 66 percent of its total calories from fat. That means that more than half of all the calories in the beef come from the fat. A Porterhouse steak contains 42 percent of its calories in fat. T-bone steak (lean), 42 percent; round steak (lean), 53 percent; ground beef (fairly lean), 64 percent; rib roast, 81 percent; sirloin steak, hipbone (lean, with fat remaining), 83 percent.

Ham contains about 74 percent of its calories in fat. Other cuts of pork range from 50 percent (shoulder, with the fat trimmed) to 74 percent (shoulder, with the fat remaining). Spareribs contain 80 percent of their calories in fat; pork sausage and bacon, both with 82 percent.

Forty-seven percent of all the calories in whole milk are from fat; most ice creams range from 50 percent to nearly 70 percent (one cup of ice cream contains 8.9 grams of fat); cheeses range from 66 percent (Swiss) to 71 percent (cheddar cheese, which has 30 milligrams of cholesterol and 6 grams of fat); blue cheese or Roquefort dressing contains 73 percent of its calories in fat; while butter derives 100 percent of its calories from fat. Egg yolks are loaded with fat, too: 79 percent of its calories coming from fat.

Remember, that all animal foods have cholesterol, too. One small three-ounce serving of beef liver, for example, contains 372 milligrams of cholesterol. A whole egg contains 64 percent of its total calories from fat (approximately 1.7 grams per egg), and an additional 274 milligrams of cholesterol. It is no wonder doctors recommend that people not eat any more than two eggs a week; two eggs equals 548 milligrams of cholesterol alone! Even the most orthodox of cardiovascular doctors will tell you that you should not have any more than 300 milligrams of cholesterol per day. To eat more than that is to put your life on the line.

Most fish contain low to moderate amounts of fat: Cod, haddock, flounder, sole, and halibut range from 3 to 11 percent.

Grains, most vegetables, and fruits have very small amounts of fat. For example, only 2 percent of all the calories provided by barley come from fat; only 4 percent of the calories derived from brown rice contain fat. Whole wheat has 5 percent of its calories from fat, while bulgur derives only 3 percent of its calories from fat.

Most vegetables are equally low. Carrots contain 4 percent of their calories from fat; broccoli, 8; celery, 5; cauliflower, 6; collards, 17; kale, 21; and winter squash, 5. Most fruits are also low in fat: apples, 9 percent; apricots, 3; cherries, 4; pears, 5; and strawberries, 11.

This is one reason why we say that grains, vegetables, and beans are so healthful: They contribute to maximum circulation of blood and oxygen to all cells of the body. There are many other reasons for their healthfulness, as the rest of this book will show. However, since grains, vegetables, beans, and fruit are all high carbohydrate foods, you can see that these foods contribute to maximum energy, blood circulation, and oxygen. Whole grains and vegetables, especially, are rich in minerals and vitamins. In other words, these foods are the basis for sound health.

Still, some fruits and vegetables contain considerable amounts of fat. Among them are olives, which derive 90 percent of their calories from fat, avocadoes, 82 percent; and coconut, 85.

Most beans have small amounts of fat—lentils have 3 percent fat; black beans, 4 percent; chick-peas (or garbanzos), 11 percent; lima beans, 4 percent. Soybeans, which derive 37 percent of their calories from fat, contain moderate amounts of fat.

However nuts are very high in fat. Peanuts derive 70 percent of their total calories from fat; almonds, 76 percent; Brazil nuts, 86 percent; macadamia nuts, 87 percent; sunflower seeds, 71 percent; walnuts, 82 percent.

High fat foods, which are the ones most commonly eaten among Western and industrialized peoples, dramatically raise blood cholesterol.

What is a safe blood cholesterol then?

From the 1950s to the early 1980s, most doctors believed that a normal cholesterol level was anywhere between 150 mg/dl to 300 mg/dl. But a U.S. government research study, called the Framingham Heart Study, which was conducted in Framingham, Massachusetts, discovered that people with cholesterol levels between 200 mg/dl to 240 mg/dl suffered from far more heart attacks than people with cholesterol levels below 180 mg/dl.

The Framingham study showed that if your cholesterol level is 200 or more, you are seriously at risk of suffering from a coronary heart attack. However, if your cholesterol level is below 180, your chances of having a heart attack are small.

Traditional people who consume very low fat and low cholesterol diets have no trouble keeping their cholesterol levels below 150 mg. Actually, a cholesterol level of 150 mg is high in China, where cholesterol levels are usually anywhere from 120 mg to 150 mg.

Nathan Pritikin—the pioneer scientist who used a whole grain and vegetable diet to treat heart disease—used to have a formula for what a safe cholesterol level should be for you. Pritikin said that your cholesterol level should be 100-plus-your-age. He said that no one's cholesterol level should exceed 160 mg, because everything above 160 mg is atherogenic, meaning that it creates atherosclerosis in the arteries throughout the body. Everything below 160 mg causes the body to eliminate atherosclerosis that has been building up inside the body. (We will talk in greater detail about reversing atherosclerosis and other illnesses later on.)

The average American cholesterol level is about 212 mg/dl, according to NHLBI. (It varies between men and women. The

average man's cholesterol is 215; the average female is about
210.) However, most men over 40 have a cholesterol level of
220 mg/dl or higher.

Research has shown that a cholesterol level below 160 mg/dl
keeps atherosclerotic plaques from forming inside the arteries.
However, a cholesterol level above 190 mg causes rapid
atherosclerosis.

These atherosclerotic plaques are like boils that develop inside
the arteries and get larger as we continue to eat high fat and high
cholesterol foods. Eventually, they close off the flow of blood
inside the artery and cause tissues that would be nourished by
that blood to suffocate and die. When a part of the heart dies,
you suffer a heart attack; when a part of the brain dies, you
suffer a stroke.

To summarize then, a safe cholesterol level is anything below
160 mg/dl. A slight margin of safety may exist between 160 mg/dl
and about 180 mg/dl, but it is wiser to keep your cholesterol
level below 160 mg to be on the safe side. Anything above 190 mg
is increasingly atherogenic—meaning that it is causing atherosclerotic plaques to form inside your arteries, especially the
coronary arteries.

From 200 mg/dl to 220 mg/dl, your risk of having a heart attack
is more than double of those whose cholesterol is below 180.
From 220 to 240, the risk is two and a half times that of 180,
and at 240 to 260 its three times the risk at 180. Cardiologists
often refer to cholesterol levels above 240 as creating "galloping
atherosclerosis," meaning that plaques are forming so rapidly
that a heart attack is almost a certainty, unless something else
kills you first.

**What is atherosclerosis and how does cholesterol in the blood
create it?**

The transformation of going from clean, healthy and un-
obstructed arteries to vessels that are closed off by bulging boils
begins with a single high fat meal. Let us say you drink a tall
glass of milk or eat a wedge of cheese or pay a visit to the "king

of coronaries," McDonald's. After you have consumed your
Big Mac, fries, and shake, tiny droplets of fat permeate your
bloodstream. These tiny microns of fat, or chylomicrons, pour
into your blood and attach themselves to your red blood cells,
causing the red cells to adhere to one another, a condition called
the *rouleaux effect,* which we described in Chapter 1. Once the
red cells are clumped together, they get stuck at the bottlenecks
to capillaries and other smaller vessels, preventing blood from
flowing to tissues throughout the body, including the brain. As
oxygen levels to the brain diminish, you begin to feel sleepy.
You want to take a nap. Your eyes feel heavy and your thought
processes become clouded. The reason your brain and eyes begin
to tire is because these two organs require much more oxygen
than the rest of the body. Consequently, any depletion in oxygen
causes the brain and eyes to react first. Long before your arms
and legs get weak, your brain gets tired and your eyes are at
half mast.

After your blood is flooded with fat and cholesterol, LDL
cholesterol heads for the walls of the artery.

Each of your arteries is layered. Each layer or sheath is composed of cells that fit together in a distinct formation, much like
a jigsaw puzzle, so that every layer of the artery has its own
jigsaw design. The innermost layer of the artery, where the blood
passes, is called the *intima*. The middle layer is called the *media*,
and the outermost layer is called the *adventitia.*

Under healthy conditions, the intima lining is clean and
smooth. However, when you eat a diet rich in fat and cholesterol, these intima cells begin to engorge themselves with particles of fat and cholesterol, or LDL, causing the cells of the
intima lining to swell. These engorged cells are now called *foam
cells* because they are swollen with cholesterol.

Scientists believe that, at this point, the cholesterol inside the
foam cells becomes rancid, or oxidize. In other words, it spoils,
as ordinary fat would spoil when left out of one's refrigerator.
In chemical terms, that spoiling, or oxidation, means that the
atom loses one or more electrons, causing the molecule to become unstable. In a stable atom, there are the same number of

negatively-charged electrons as there are positively-charged protons. But when the cholesterol oxidizes, the atoms begin to lose electrons, causing the molecules to break down and decay.

This instability is an unhealthy or foreign condition, and causes the immune system to respond. Macrophage cells, which are immune cells that gobble up bacteria, pathogens, and other foreign invaders, rush to the artery wall and begin to ingest the rancid cholesterol. These macrophage cells become trapped inside the artery wall. They swell with cholesterol and become foam cells themselves.

These foam cells form clusters, or what is called a *fatty streak*—a yellow streak inside the artery. This fatty streak is the early stage of an atherosclerotic lesion, or plaque. The cells themselves have chemicals within them that could rid themselves of the cholesterol and eliminate the fatty streak—if the person stopped eating a diet rich in fat and cholesterol. However, that usually does not happen. Consequently, the problem only gets worse.

As more cholesterol floods the bloodstream and is carried to the wall of the artery by LDL, the fatty streak grows. More intima cells inside the artery consume the LDL; more macrophage cells hurry to the area and become foam cells themselves; consequently, the lesions become larger. It grows in both directions—up, into the passageway of the artery, and down, into the next layer of the artery wall, the media. As the plaque grows, it ultimately threatens to close off the passageway of the artery.

Blood infuses these plaques, along with calcium and fiber. The arrival of calcium and fiber causes the plaque to have a hard, pearly cap on top of it. This fibrous cap seals off the boil from the blood traveling inside the artery. However, blood does reach the interior of the artery, because the body forms new blood vessels that travel through the outermost lining of the artery, the adventitia, and into the media level. Now blood is flowing from the other direction of the artery wall. Since that blood contains LDL cholesterol, too, the atherosclerotic process continues, which makes the plaque larger.

Ultimately, part of these plaques can break off and flow to the heart and cause a heart attack. Even if the plaque does not break off, it can grow so large that it can block blood from flowing to a particular part of the body. If it is growing inside the coronary artery, blood will stop flowing to the heart, which will cause part of the heart muscle to suffocate and die, a condition typically referred to as a heart attack.

If blood stops flowing to the brain, a part of the brain will die and the person will suffer a stroke. As everyone knows, a heart attack or stroke can be fatal; it can also be severely debilitating.

But atherosclerosis is taking place elsewhere in the body as well. For example, many people have plaque clogging the vessels and arteries of the legs. This prevents optimal amounts of oxygen from flowing to the leg muscles. When a person with this condition takes a walk, he often feels great pain in his legs, a condition called *claudication*. The problem is that the diminished blood flow is not bringing adequate amounts of oxygen to the muscles. In addition, the blood is not removing lactic acid from the muscles, which builds up during exercise. The increased acid and decreased oxygen cause great pain, which requires the person to rest so that the blood flow can remove the acid content of the muscles and bring more oxygen.

How is diet related to blood pressure?

High blood pressure, or hypertension as it is also called, is the most common cardiovascular illness in the United States. It is an important risk factor in the development of atherosclerosis, and leads to both heart attack and stroke. Many people have high blood pressure, but do not know it. Like many other forms of heart disease, such as atherosclerosis, high blood pressure often has no overt symptoms. Nevertheless, it can lead to kidney damage, pancreatic disease, and disorders of the eye. High blood pressure often results in aneurysms, or "blowouts," of arteries leading to the brain; the result is a stroke.

Blood pressure is considered high when it exceeds 140/90. Many insurers will not carry a policy on someone when the lower number of the blood pressure scale exceeds 85.

Blood pressure is caused by the expansion and contraction of the heart. The diastolic phase occurs when the heart relaxes and opens, and allows blood to flow into the chambers. The systolic phase occurs when the heart contracts, causing blood to be pumped through the arterial system and throughout the body.

Blood pressure increases with age in the United States and much of the Western world, but in pre-modern societies and places that still follow traditional diets, blood pressure tends to remain within the healthy range throughout life. Contrary to what many people believe, elevated blood pressure is not an inevitable consequence of aging.

There are three main causes of high blood pressure: athero-sclerosis, excessive salt intake, and kidney disease.

Atherosclerosis raises blood pressure by narrowing the passage-way within arteries. This causes pressure to build behind the blood that is backed up. The effect is analogous to pinching a hose to increase the pressure of the water that flows out.

Excessive salt intake causes edema, which increases the plasma or liquid portion of the blood. Greater quantities of plasma mean increased blood flow within arteries and veins that have distinct limits. Salt also causes the tiny renal arteries in kidneys to con-tract, which causes blood to back up behind the kidneys and thus increases pressure.

We encourage people to use good quality sea salt in cooking and to add small portions of *tamari* soy sauce (*shoyu*) and *miso* and other fermented products to the diet (see recipe and menu sections for details). Sea salt, tamari soy sauce, and miso alkalize food, making it easier to digest. Food is alkalized by chewing— which infuses it with saliva, an alkaline substance. It is also alkalized by the presence of minerals, such as sodium, zinc, selenium, calcium, magnesium, manganese, and others (see Chapter 8). Minerals are essential to a healthy functioning immune system. Sea salt, and the salt found in miso and tamari soy sauce, also opens up the grain, making it easier to chew and digest. Finally, good quality sea salt contains trace minerals not found in sodium chloride or normal table salt.

Of course, salt is a substance we must be careful with, as well. We want to use small amounts of salt. Too much can cause high blood pressure and kidney disorders. In most cases tamari soy sauce and miso should not be added to food at the table, but only used in cooking.

Because these fermented foods contain friendly digestive bacteria, they should not be boiled when used in cooking, which would kill the bacteria. (See cooking instructions.)

You can lower blood pressure simply by reducing the amount of fat in your diet. In most cases, blood pressure will be reduced, even if salt is kept at a constant. However, we do not recommend using high quantities of salt. People with high blood pressure should reduce both fat and salt in the diet. They will see a rapid decline in their blood pressure within a matter of weeks.

In 1974, Dr. Frank Sacks of the Harvard Medical School studied the blood pressures of 210 people following a macrobiotic diet. His research showed that the average blood pressure among these macrobiotic people was 106/60, very low, and very healthy. In his published report (*American Journal of Epidemiology*, Vol. 100; No. 5), Dr. Sacks noted that "Epidemiological surveys [population studies] . . . show a trend linking diets containing little meat and fish to low mean blood pressures . . . ." The macrobiotic diet, Dr. Sacks stated, is low in animal foods; fish is the most consistent animal food consumed. Consequently, the low blood pressures of those on the macrobiotic diet is consistent with the blood pressures of populations around the world where the diets are made up mainly of whole grains, beans, vegetables, fruit, and fish.

I thought oat bran lowered cholesterol. Now I hear that it does not do anything. What is the truth?

Back in the 1970s and early 1980s researchers discovered that soluble fiber, found in such foods as oats and brown rice, lowered cholesterol level. Initially, the studies seemed convincing, especially the research done by Dr. James Anderson at the University of Kentucky Medical School, who used soluble fiber—along with a low fat and cholesterol diet—to lower cholesterol and aid in the treatment of adult-onset diabetes. (We will discuss the role of fat and cholesterol in the onset and reversal of adult-onset diabetes in Chapter 5 of this book.)

Later research, done by Dr. Jeremiah Stamler at Northwestern University Medical School showed that the average person needed to eat 35 grams of oat bran cereal (about 2/3 of a cup, cooked) to lower his cholesterol level by 3 percent.

This resulted in an explosion of oat bran commercials and oat bran marketing. Oat bran was suddenly being referred to as "oat cuisine," replacing haute cuisine, and put into everything from cereals to breads, muffins, potato chips, popcorn, and cookies.

But was it really working? Two studies published in January 1990—one done by Brigham and Women's Hospital in Boston and the other at Syracuse University—both answered "No." The studies demonstrated that oat bran was not independently lowering cholesterol to any significant degree. Any cholesterol lowering that did take place resulted from the fact that oats and oat bran are low in fat and cholesterol, and that this food was crowding out high fat foods from the diet.

Dr. Frank Sacks, Harvard University researcher who conducted the Brigham and Women's Hospital study, said, "What we knew 25 years ago about reducing cholesterol is what we know now, and there's not much new under the sun. Saturated fat and cholesterol are paramount."

Sacks pointed out that oat bran did not lower cholesterol any better than refined wheat flour (common white flour). The reason cholesterol was lowered at all was because oat bran was being "substituted" for foods that were high in fat and cholesterol. For example, if you ate an oat bran breakfast, you were probably not eating eggs and bacon, both of which are high in fat and cholesterol. This would naturally result in a lowered cholesterol level. That phenomenon had previously been attributed to oat bran alone, but according to Sacks the same cholesterol lowering would have occurred if one had eaten, say, dry rye toast.

After these two studies were reported, researchers around the country called for more research, which is a common outcry among scientists, especially where there is controversy. The question suddenly facing many people was: Should I go on eating oat bran?

The answer is an unequivocal "No." The only sure way to lower your cholesterol level is to substantially reduce the saturated fat and cholesterol in your diet. If you eat a diet rich in meat, eggs, chicken, and dairy products, your cholesterol level will skyrocket—no matter how much oat bran you eat in addition. That goes for omega-3 polyunsaturated fish oils, as well.

People who insist on eating high fat foods are always hoping for a magic bullet. Many researchers, pharmaceutical and food companies prey on this hope by offering the latest in cholesterol-lowering supplements or drugs. The supplements will not make much difference in your cholesterol level, however, and the drugs have side effects, some of them severe.

The best way for you to improve your overall health, including lowering your cholesterol level, is to adopt the dietary guidelines offered in this book. That will ensure a lower cholesterol level, as well as many other health benefits. We must deal with our cholesterol levels as a symptom of our overall health. The quality of our blood is a reflection of what we eat. To eat a high fat diet and consume lots of supplements, such as oat bran or fish oils, is to live like a house divided. What we are really saying is that we want to do as we please with impunity, which is, as we all know, against the laws of the universe. If you consume a diet rich in fat and cholesterol, you will need drugs and possibly surgery to deal with your sicknesses, because the supplements will not be sufficient to eliminate the consequences of your diet.

Do you recommend any supplements?

In general, "No."

Within the body, there is a unity or an integrity that causes the body to function as a whole. The body has been referred to as an ecosystem, in which all the parts are participating together—much as individual instruments combine to bring forth a symphony. The liver is absolutely dependent upon the healthy functioning of the kidneys; the kidneys depend on the healthy functioning of the large intestine and lungs; the lungs on the spleen and stomach; the spleen on the heart and small intestine. The body works as a orchestra, each organ interacting and blending with the others to bring forth harmony and efficient function.

The evolution of the human body, which has taken place over two million years, cannot be separated from its experience of food, particularly the food humans have depended upon the most: grains and vegetables. Our bodies have evolved and adapted to the vegetable kingdom. We have literally been shaped and structured so that we can eat whole, vegetable foods. It is for this reason that we have thirty-two teeth and a long digestive tract.

When we examine our teeth, we notice that we have twenty molars and premolars, perfect for grinding grains and vegetables. We also have eight incisors, which are perfect for biting off vegetables and bread (or grain products). Only four of our teeth are canine, whose purpose is to tear flesh, or help us consume animal foods. If you look at the teeth of a dog, you see a mouth full of canine teeth. Evolution has equipped the dog, cat, lion, and tiger with the perfect set of teeth for flesh eating. Human teeth reveal an essential truth: that the human diet should be composed chiefly of vegetable foods, such as grains, leafy greens, beans, carrots, fruits, and many others.

Unlike carnivores, humans are also blessed with long digestive tracts, which are ideal for digesting whole grains and vegetables, but less than ideal for consuming animal foods. Grains and vegetables are composed chiefly of complex carbohydrates, which require greater exposure to enzymes within the digestive tract in order to be transformed into glucose, or blood sugar used as a fuel for cells. Simple carbohydrates, found in refined sugar, make their way into the bloodstream the minute they touch the tongue, and consequently cause blood sugar levels to rise quickly. That fuel is also burned quickly, causing blood sugar levels to fall as fast as they rose. This is the reason refined sugars give rise to feelings of weakness and lethargy, a disease known as hypoglycemia. Whole grains, on the other hand, burn slowly and provide steady energy flow and long-term endurance.

Animal foods require short digestive tracts—the kind you see in dogs, cats, lions, and tigers—because the fat in animal foods quickly becomes rancid and gives rise to free radicals (explained in Chapter 1), ammonia, and other toxins that cause cancer, heart disease, and other illnesses. Animal foods need to be digested and eliminated quickly. For that, you need a short digestive tract. (See Chapter 5 for an explanation of colon cancer.)

You can see that there is a marvelous consistency between human teeth and the human digestive system. The teeth and the digestive tract suggest that our diets should be made up primarily of whole vegetable foods, with smaller portions of animal foods, if desired.

Moreover, the very presence of our teeth and digestive tract suggest that we naturally draw our nutrition from *food*—not from pills. Our bodies have evolved and adapted to food. We are used to extracting nutrients from whole foods in digestion. Food provides combinations of nutrients with which bodies are familiar and upon which we are dependent. Supplementation creates imbalances of specific nutrients, many of which are harmful in high quantities. For years, people took brewer's yeast thinking it was healthful, only to find out later that it created candidiasis. Excess consumption of iron, vitamin A, and many other nutrients are toxic.

Putting nutrients in pill form is an altogether recent phenomenon. This separation of nutrients from their original state makes the nutrients themselves foreign to human biology and evolution. Combinations of nutrients exist in whole foods that cannot be found in pills.

The act of taking nutrition involves our direct connection to nature. Food experiences the cycles of nature, the daily path of the sun, the changing weather patterns, the characteristics of the air, soil, and water. Food is therefore the product of nature, and as such it embodies the events and influences of the environment.

By eating food, we become one with nature. By preparing food and eating it—that is, the act of cooking, chewing, tasting, digesting, assimilating nutrients and eliminating what we do not need—we are deeply experiencing nature. If we grow that food, too, it is all the better, because our relationship with the vegetable kingdom becomes even deeper.

Moreover, whole foods address the needs of a whole person. Grain, for example, provides carbohydrates for energy, protein for cell replacement and repair; vitamins and minerals for metabolism; small amounts of fat for reserves of energy; and fiber to assist digestion and elimination. Whole grains meet the needs of the whole human being.

When looked at in this way, we see that getting proper nutrition is more than simply adding up our vitamins and minerals. It is our basic human link with the mother of life on the planet: nature herself.

Let us talk about the effects of the common high fat and high cholesterol diet on the cardiovascular system. What is the risk?

The diet most of us consume in the West—rich in fat, cholesterol, sugar, and artificial ingredients—is causing an epidemic of unmatched proportion. According to the American Heart Association, 66 million Americans suffer from illnesses of the heart and arteries, collectively known as *cardiovascular disease*. These illnesses include coronary heart disease, stroke, and high blood pressure. One million Americans die every year from such illnesses, which amounts to half of all deaths in the U.S.

Coronary heart disease afflicts 5 million people and kills half a million annually. High blood pressure, or hypertension, afflicts 60 million Americans, thousands of whom are children and teenagers. Almost half of all people with high blood pressure do not even know they have the disease. More than 30,000 die annually from the illness.

Five hundred thousand people each year suffer a stroke. Of these, approximately 150,000 die.

Nearly 50 million Americans have blood cholesterol levels of

240 mg/dl, and nearly 100 million have cholesterol levels of 200 mg/dl or better.

The cost of cardiovascular disease is staggering—nearly $100 billion a year is spent on medical care (including doctors, nurses, and medication), hospital bills, and lost wages.

A lot of this money goes to surgery, specifically coronary bypass surgery. Three-hundred-and-fifty-thousand coronary artery bypass surgeries are performed annually, the majority of them (about 70 percent) on men, at a cost of about $20,000 a piece, depending on the number of coronary arteries replaced in the surgery.

You would think that all of this would be enough to generate a national alert and radically change our eating habits, but such changes are slow in coming, and many people, including doctors and scientists, do not believe the evidence exists to make such changes.

Let us have a look at an overview of that evidence.

At the turn of the century, Sir William Osler, a British researcher, had found that atherosclerosis—an illness in which cholesterol plaques form inside the walls of arteries—was far more common among the British aristocracy than among the poor. Osler theorized that the diet of the rich might be the cause of the atherosclerosis because the rich ate rich and fatty foods, while the poor ate mostly grains and vegetables, foods that were low in fat and free of cholesterol.

A few decades later, a Russian scientist by the name of Nikolai Anitschow reported in 1913 that rabbits fed meat, eggs, and milk developed high degrees of atherosclerosis and heart disease. Those rabbits that were fed vegetables did not get atherosclerosis and heart disease.

During World War II, several European nations rationed such foods as butter, meat, eggs, and cheese from the civilian population and sent them to their soldiers fighting the war. These foods were thought to be the most nutritious available, and therefore vital to the health and strength of the fighting men. Consequently, the civilian population was forced to revert to its "peasant" diet, made up largely of whole grains, such as wheat, barley, corn, and rice; potatoes and other vegetables; and fruits. During the war years, the death rate from heart disease among civilians in countries that were food rationed dropped dramatically.

Dr. William Castelli, director of the Framingham Heart Study, the largest on-going heart disease study in the world, was a young medical intern in Belgium during the war and watched the heart disease rate among civilians plummet. Said Castelli: "There wasn't enough atherosclerosis in the coronary arteries of those people to show medical school students what it looked like." Atherosclerosis is the underlying cause of most heart attacks, strokes, and high blood pressure.

In 1956, a Japanese physician, Dr. N. Kimura, compared the autopsy records of 10,000 Japanese war dead with American soldiers killed during the war and found that the Japanese had a marked absence of atherosclerosis, while their American counterparts had significant and even advanced heart disease.

Later, the famed Ancel Keyes examined populations of seven countries—some 12,000 people—and found that where the diets were high in fat and cholesterol, there was a higher incidence of heart disease and other serious illnesses.

Autopsies done on Americans killed during the Korean and Vietnam wars showed significant artery closure among half of the men killed, whose average age was 22.

In China, where heart disease is rare and life expectancy exceeds 70 years, a low cholesterol level is anywhere from 90 mg/dl to 120 mg/dl. It is rare to find a cholesterol level above 150.

Scientists also found that Japanese who remained in Japan rarely suffered from heart disease, cancer, adult-onset diabetes, and other serious degenerative diseases. However, when they migrated to the United States, their rates of heart disease, cancer, and other illnesses rose to American levels. In Japan, an adult's cholesterol level is usually below 150 mg/dl. The Japanese have the lowest heart attack rate in the world, about one-fourth that of the United States. But when Japanese come to the United States and adopt an American diet, their cholesterol levels go up to 200 mg/dl and higher; their rates of heart disease reach American levels, as well.

The Framingham Heart Study has followed the people of Framingham, Massachusetts since 1948 and demonstrated conclusively that as blood cholesterol levels rise, so, too, does the incidence of heart attacks and strokes.

The Finns eat a diet that is richer in fat and cholesterol than anywhere else in the world. They also have the highest cholesterol levels, and the highest heart disease rate, as well. The second highest heart disease rate is the United States's.

Laboratory studies have demonstrated over and over again that a high fat and high cholesterol diet raises blood cholesterol levels and dramatically increases the rate of heart diseases.

In January, 1984, the National Heart, Lung and Blood Institute announced that after a ten year study involving 3,000 men, at a cost of $150 million, scientists had proven conclusively that a high fat and high cholesterol diet does indeed cause heart disease. The study demonstrated that by lowering the fat and cholesterol in the diet, people can reduce their chances of suffering from a heart attack, or some other form of cardiovascular disease. The scientists went so far as to say that a 1 percent drop in blood cholesterol equalled a 2 percent drop in your chances of suffering a heart attack. By cutting cholesterol level by 25 percent, you could cut your chances of having a heart attack in half. (As we will show in the next chapter, other studies demonstrated conclusively that by lowering your cholesterol level, you could reverse atherosclerosis, the underlying cause of heart disease.)

These studies and many others were too much to ignore. After this mountain of research, politicians and scientists began to publish dietary recommendations, acknowledging that the typical high fat and high cholesterol diet was the cause of most of our modern ills. *Dietary Goals for the United States*, published in 1977 by the Senate Select Committee on Nutrition and Human Needs, stated unequivocally that six-out-of-the-ten leading causes of death were directly related to the American diet. These illnesses included heart disease, cancer, diabetes, high blood pressure, obesity, and liver disease. *Dietary Goals* recommended that Americans reduce their consumption of foods high in fat, cholesterol, sugar, salt, and artificial ingredients, and increase their consumption of whole grains, fresh vegetables, fruit, and fish.

Dietary Goals was followed by reports by the U.S. Surgeon General, the U.S. Departments of Agriculture and Health, Education, and Welfare (now called Health and Human Services), and the National Research Council, all urging Americans to change their ways of eating to reduce the risk of disease.

Despite what some scientists and doctors would have you believe, there is an overwhelming consensus on the relationship between diet and health. That consensus is that a high fat and high cholesterol diet causes illness, especially heart disease and cancer. To turn your back on such information is, literally, risking your life.

Health is a birthright; the truth has always been with us.

The knowledge of how diet effects health has always been available. It is just the forms of that knowledge that have changed. Throughout history, the understanding of how diet affects health has existed in two forms: as traditional and philosophical teachings, and as scientific research. These two sources of information represent parallel schools, from which healers, teachers, and physicians have derived their knowledge. Of course, the traditional and philosophical knowledge has been around the longest. *The Yellow Emperor's Classic of Internal Medicine*—regarded today as the oldest medical book in existence—was written some 2,500 years ago by Chinese sages. Western scientific research is a good deal younger. Good evidence that certain diets cause serious illness and other diets foster health was available in the early 1900s.

Even in the 1950s, there were sufficient puzzle pieces available to see the picture, if they were put together properly. But you had to be a really good detective to put the pieces together and very few people were able to do it. Only a handful of people actually managed it. Those few included George Ohsawa, who is the modern inventor of macrobiotics; Michio Kushi, who was one of Ohsawa's principal students; and Nathan Pritikin, who invented the Pritikin Program. The macrobiotic and Pritikin diets were created on the basis of traditional cultures—that is, cultures where modern technology had not interfered with the traditional ways of eating.

Ohsawa gained his understanding from the Chinese and Japanese writings. Born in 1893, Ohsawa contracted tuberculosis when he was 18 years old. His physicians informed Ohsawa and his mother that his disease was incurable. However, Ohsawa encountered the writings of the nineteenth century physician Sagen Ishizuka, who used a diet of brown rice, vegetables, beans, sea vegetables, and sea salt to treat serious illnesses. Ohsawa followed Sagen's advice and cured himself. Afterward, he made the study of diet and health a lifelong passion. It was Sagen's writings that introduced Ohsawa to *The Yellow Emperor's Classic of Internal Medicine*, which formed the foundation of much of his knowledge of diet and health. Ohsawa's understanding of food's influence on life went so deeply that it touched every aspect of human existence. He saw food's connection to physical, psychological, and spiritual development. Ohsawa joined the writings of Sagen and the Yellow Emperor with the underlying traditional philosophy of the Orient and called his overall view "macrobiotics," meaning big or great life. He passed his knowledge on to Kushi and other students, including Herman Aihara, another important teacher of macrobiotics. These and other people developed Ohsawa's understanding even further and spread the teachings of macrobiotics around the world.

When historians of the twenty-first century look back at this period of history, they are going to marvel at how we managed to miss the obvious. They will also recognize the consequences of our ignorance.

What if I lower my cholesterol level? Can I get my health back?

Yes. But you will have to turn to the next chapter to understand how.

Chapter 3

Curing Atherosclerosis and Heart Disease: "True Facts"

In the spring of 1982, Lew Ross weighed 220 pounds. At five-feet-eight-inches, the forty-year-old Ross was 70 pounds over-weight. That was only one of his problems. He was borderline diabetic, and suffered from tremors, severe stomach pains, insomnia, and illnesses of the gallbladder, liver, kidneys, and pancreas. He was chronically depressed; he was also an alcoholic. Ross's doctors had prescribed Lithium, Triavil, and Ludimil for the depression, and Restorild for the insomnia, but the drugs were causing side effects and were not as effective as Lew would have liked. Blood tests revealed that Ross's cholesterol level was 383 mg/dl.

In the late summer of that year, Lew Ross visited his doctor, hoping to get even more medication for his growing list of diseases. Once his doctor took his blood pressure, however, he simply sat back and looked at Ross in shock. Ross's blood pressure was 175/125. His blood pressure and cholesterol level were so frighteningly high that a heart attack or stroke seemed imminent.

"I don't know what to say, Mr. Ross," the doctor said. "There is nothing else I can do for you."

Shaken by his doctor's grave tone, Ross pressed the physician to give him more drugs.

"No," the doctor said flatly. "There are no more drugs that can help you."

Ross was instructed not to exert himself, lest he bring on a fatal stroke or heart attack. The picture his physician was draw-ing for him was painfully clear: at the age of forty, Lew Ross could not expect to live much longer.

A resident of Washington, D.C., Ross knew a fellow employee

at Pan American Airlines who was practicing a macrobiotic diet and had made a remarkable improvement in her health. Ross asked the woman about the diet and lifestyle and, after listening to the woman, decided he would investigate it further.

Lew Ross went back to his doctor and asked him if he knew anything about macrobiotics. The doctor said that based on the little he knew of macrobiotics, he felt confident that it would do Ross good to adopt the diet. In talking to his doctor, Ross got the impression that the diet might be his last hope.

Ross did adopt the diet. He saw macrobiotic counselor Michael Rossoff in Washington for advice on beginning macrobiotics, and thus began a miraculous journey back to health.

Once on the diet, Lew Ross lost 20 pounds a month, yet ate at least three large meals per day and never went hungry.

"People were amazed at how much I could eat, and yet I was losing weight rapidly," Ross recalled. In the months that followed, Ross's weight dropped from 220 to 135 pounds. From there, it crept back up to an optimal 149, where it has stayed ever since.

His weight loss was only one of the benefits of the diet, however. Ross's cholesterol level dropped from 383 mg/dl to 141 mg/dl. His blood pressure fell to 110/70, both medically ideal. Other tests showed that his liver, kidney, pancreas, and gallbladder functions had been restored to health.

In addition, Ross's energy levels, outlook on life, and clarity of mind dramatically improved. His appearance went from an obese body and glazed skin, to a trim, fit body, and bright and clean complexion.

Gradually, Rossoff helped Ross wean himself from all medication. With the aid of a "Twelve Step" alcohol rehabilitation program, Ross also eliminated alcohol from his life.

Within three years of beginning the diet, Ross was a new man. As far as he was concerned, he had experienced a miracle.

Ross's story is significant for many reasons. Among them is the fact that like many overweight people he suffered from a variety of illnesses, including heart disease, high blood pressure, and diabetes. His underlying illness was food poisoning, however.

Fat and cholesterol, sugar and other refined foods combined to overwhelm his system. He might have died from a heart attack or stroke. But the real problem in his life was his diet. And no drug in the world could cure that. As with many people who come to macrobiotics, Ross experienced a general rejuvenation. It was not just his weight or high blood pressure or cholesterol level that was affected, but every aspect of his health—indeed, everything in his life.

That is a very exciting case history, but you said that the macrobiotic diet, if used properly, could reverse atherosclerosis. How do you know that is happening?

Let us begin with the proof that diet and lifestyle alone can reverse atherosclerosis, and then proceed to describe how it can be done.

In November 1989, Dr. Dean Ornish, director of the Preventive Medicine Research Institute in Sausalito, California, reported a study showing reversal of atherosclerosis in the coronary arteries of humans on a low fat and low cholesterol diet. Ornish's research, which was reported at the annual meeting of the American Heart Association, is the first study to show that diet and lifestyle alone can reverse atherosclerosis in the coronary arteries in humans. Unlike other studies that demonstrated reversal, Ornish's study used no cholesterol-lowering drugs.

Ornish enlisted the cooperation of forty-eight men and women, all of whom had coronary artery disease and were scheduled for angiograms, a test used to determine the amount of atherosclerosis clogging the coronary arteries. All forty-eight people showed significant closure of the coronary arteries after their angiograms.

These forty-eight people were divided into two groups of twenty-four each. One group was given the standard medical advice for heart disease: they were encouraged to adopt a 30 percent fat diet, stop smoking, and do aerobic exercise three times per week. This group was called the control group.

The experimental group was placed on a vegetarian diet that

derived only 8 percent of its calories from fat. The foods that the experimental group ate were primarily whole grains and vegetables. They also received instruction in stress management, performed yoga and aerobic exercise. All of the members of the experimental group stopped smoking, as well.

The two groups were followed for one year. Before they began receiving their treatment, the average blood cholesterol level in the experimental group was 213 mg/dl. However, after they adopted their low fat and low cholesterol diet, their cholesterol levels fell to an average of 154 mg/dl.

The control group started out with an average cholesterol level of 251 mg/dl, and managed to bring that down to 230 on the 30 percent fat diet.

After one year, angiograms were performed once again on the remaining participants of both groups. (Seven had dropped out of the study, two from the experimental group and five from the control group. Interestingly, compliance was better among the experimental group than the controls, who received the less demanding program.)

Of the twenty-two remaining participants in the experimental group, eighteen members showed reversal of atherosclerosis in the coronary arteries. That is, the atherosclerotic plaque in the arteries leading to the heart got smaller, making the passageway within the artery larger.

In the control group, ten of the remaining nineteen members showed a worsening of the atherosclerotic plaque. Three members remained the same, and six got slightly better.

After reviewing the study, Dr. Claude L'Enfant, director of the National Heart, Lung and Blood Institute, stated: "I feel this is a tremendously important study in the control of coronary artery disease without pharmaceutical intervention."

Dr. R. Lance Gould, cardiologist at the Center for Cardiology and Imaging Research at the University of Texas Medical School in Houston, told *The New York Times* that, "This proves you can reverse heart disease without drugs if you take the lifestyle far enough."

Reversal of atherosclerosis in the coronary arteries of humans had been demonstrated by Dr. David Blankenhorn and his colleagues at the University of Southern California. However, Blankenhorn used drugs to lower the blood cholesterol of his patients. Dean Ornish's study did it by diet and lifestyle alone.

He did it by getting the cholesterol level of his patients down just below 160 mg/dl.

For many years, reversal of atherosclerosis had been shown in rhesus monkeys, most notably at the University of Chicago where Dr. Robert Wissler placed monkeys on a high fat diet, watched their cholesterol levels increase dramatically, and recorded the consequent growth of atherosclerosis. He then placed the same monkeys on a diet low in fat and cholesterol and demonstrated reversal of atherosclerosis. Within eighteen months, the coronary arteries of the monkeys were clean again.

M. L. Armstrong had performed the same study on rhesus monkeys with the same results in 1970. He conducted other studies comparing specific kinds of diets. In one study, Armstrong placed thirty monkeys on a high fat, high cholesterol diet for nearly a year-and-a-half. At that point, ten animals were examined to see the extent of atherosclerosis that was blocking their coronary arteries and found that the arteries were more than 50 percent closed due to plaque. This group of ten monkeys he called the baseline group.

He then placed ten of the remaining animals on a no-cholesterol, low fat diet. The other ten he placed on a diet of no-cholesterol, but high in *unsaturated* fat. He wanted to see what effect the unsaturated fat would have on the coronary atherosclerosis.

After forty months, Armstrong examined the coronary arteries of both groups of animals. The monkeys on the no-cholesterol, low fat diet had experienced a dramatic reversal of coronary atherosclerosis: their plaques were now one fourth the size of the original baseline group on the high fat, high cholesterol diet. In other words, they had experienced a 75 percent reversal of atherosclerosis in just over three years. The monkeys on the no-cholesterol, high unsaturated fat diet had also experienced reversal of atherosclerosis, but not to the degree of the no-cholesterol, low fat group. The high unsaturated fat group experienced only half the reversal of the low fat group.

Armstrong's research showed that the diet that was most effective at reversing coronary atherosclerosis was low in cholesterol and all fats.

The key to reversing atherosclerosis is lowering blood cholesterol below 160 mg/dl. Once you get your cholesterol down below that level, your body will be able to eliminate the atherosclerotic plaque that is clogging your arteries. However, once you get your cholesterol down below 160, you have to keep it there in order to benefit. Atherosclerosis takes time to reverse and can easily come back if your cholesterol level climbs again.

Getting your cholesterol down below 160 mg/dl seems very difficult. I have read in popular magazines that people cannot stick to low fat diets and therefore they are not really beneficial.

Many doctors and scientists have argued that you cannot get a free-living population of people to lower their cholesterol level significantly and keep it low. They argue that in order to lower cholesterol and keep it under control, you have got to put people in the hospital or some other clinical setting where their diets can be controlled. This is untrue, however.

In 1975, the *New England Journal of Medicine* (May 29, 1975; 292: 1148–1151) published a study done by Drs. Frank Sacks, William Castelli, and their associates which found that a population of free-living macrobiotic people had extremely low cholesterol levels.

Seventy-three men and forty-three women who followed the macrobiotic diet agreed to participate in the study. They were randomly selected from a larger population of macrobiotic people living in the greater Boston area. On the average, the 116 men and women had been practicing macrobiotics three years. Another group of men and women were also randomly selected and matched according to age and sex. This group was called the control group, and would be used to compare the cholesterol levels with the macrobiotic group.

Dr. Sacks reported that the average blood cholesterol for those following the macrobiotic diet was 126 mg/dl. The average cholesterol level for the controls was 184 mg/dl.

After examining the blood cholesterol levels of the macrobiotic people, Dr. Sacks wrote: "Levels of plasma lipids [blood fats and cholesterol] in the [macrobiotic] group were found to be strikingly low in all age groups, and the rise of lipid values with age was slight."

Dr. Sacks concluded that the composition of the diet, especially its lack of animal foods, was responsible for the low cholesterol levels of the macrobiotic group.

"Overall consumption of animal products was directly related to the level of total cholesterol," wrote Dr. Sacks.

Based on the work done by Dean Ornish, whose group's average cholesterol level dropped only to 154 mg/dl, it is safe to assume that those following the macrobiotic diet were experiencing reversal of any atherosclerosis that had developed prior to their starting the macrobiotic diet.

It is important to point out that the people in the macrobiotic group had jobs, carried on normal lives, and simply agreed to have their cholesterol levels checked by the scientists. They also filled out dietary questionnaries at the request of Dr. Sacks and his colleagues. These questionnaries revealed that although the macrobiotic people did occasionally cheat from their regimens, they were remarkably consistent in their eating habits. In other words, they had no trouble sticking to the diet.

This was not the only macrobiotic group that had low cholesterol levels.

In 1980, eleven staff members of *East West Journal*, all of whom practiced macrobiotics, decided to have their cholesterol levels checked. The decision came after the staff began an issue dedicated to heart disease. All eleven staff members lived separately and followed the macrobiotic diet according to their own judgment and food choices. Their average age was thirty. The blood tests of the eleven staff members revealed that their average cholesterol level was 121 mg/dl. The range ran from a low of 102 mg/dl to a high of 147 mg/dl. Most of the staff had cholesterol levels below 115 mg/dl. All had been following the macrobiotic diet for at least two years. Moreover, all of them had eaten the typical American diet of meat, dairy products, eggs, and sugar before adopting the macrobiotic regimen.

Why are people who follow macrobiotics able to stick to the diet?

There are many reasons why macrobiotics can be followed more consistently than other diets. Among them is the fact that after a short while on the diet, you feel stronger, more vital, and more energetic. Your clarity of thought increases. You tend to sleep better and wake up more refreshed. In other words, there are rewards in the short term; you have proof that the diet is making a difference early in your practice.

Once you begin eating macrobiotically, you also develop a greater sensitivity to foods and their effects on you. For example, people feel the strong effects of sugar after they have avoided it for a while. The same is true of other foods. Consequently, you no longer need the more extreme foods—sugar, meat, eggs, and dairy products—that you ate in the past.

There is another important reason people stick to macrobiotics, however. Macrobiotics is more than a diet, but a way of understanding life, health, and illness. People come to macrobiotics not only for the diet, but for its underlying philosophy.

To put that philosophy in a nutshell, we can say that macrobiotics views all reality as the by-product of two forces, one an expansive force called *yin*, the other a contractive force, called *yang*. These forces influence all phenomena—from your personal food cravings, to your relationships with other people. Yin and yang are implicit in the changes that take place within nations and the movements of heavenly bodies. In other words, yin and yang are everywhere, from the most specific aspects of your life, to the most abstract.

These opposite forces take shape in daily life as man and woman, day and night, near and far, hot and cold, north and south, east and west, up and down, left and right. Three-dimensional reality would be impossible without opposites. All dimension is made possible by opposites.

Man and woman, or opposite sexes, make up the human race

and make procreation possible. The opposites within a twenty-four hour period—day and night—make up a full day.

Yin and yang represent opposing poles, such as the poles of a magnet. Consequently, they are always attracting each other. In this way, they create movement. Electricity is an example of the movement of energy that is made possible by opposing magnetic poles.

The seasons, for example, are an example of stages of yin and yang. Winter is the most yin season. It is more still, quiet, a time when nature rests. Summer is the most yang season: nature bursts forth with all the richness of the earth and sun.

By attracting each other, yin and yang are continually changing into the other. For example, winter—the most yin season—ultimately changes into the most yang—summer.

It is the same with daily life. We are active all day long—the yang state—but sleep at night, the yin state.

Long before there were blood tests and X ray machines and nutrient compositions of foods, traditional peoples developed an understanding of healing, food and health that was as effective as anything we have today in modern medicine. They treated all diseases. What is more, they put tremendous emphasis on preventing serious illness through the use of correct diet and life conditions.

Prevention of illness was accomplished by maintaining balance in daily eating and activity. Behavior could be understood in terms of yin and yang. Work, for example, is yang; rest is yin. Too much work will make one miserable and sick; too much rest will make one equally miserable and sick. Socializing can be seen as yin, or expansive, since you encounter greater number of people, enjoy a more diverse range of information emanating from those people, and participate vicariously in more lives than simply your own. A yang, or active, person is drawn to social activities. A yin person, or one who likes to be alone, is not drawn to the yin effects of socializing. They are drawn instead to the more yang, solitary life, because their yin nature needs that kind of life for balance and harmony. No matter how yin or yang you may be, however, too much socializing can make your life chaotic (yin), and lead to sickness. Therefore, balance between social life and time spent alone is more appropriate to maintain health.

Food can also be seen as forms of yin and yang. Yin foods have an expansive effect on the body. They make the body cool, more relaxed, and slower moving. Yang foods make the body more contracted, warmer, and more active.

In ancient times, this system of classification of foods became very specific; certain foods were used to treat specific organs, for example. Consequently, food was looked at as medicine. Hippocrates, the father of medicine, urged people to "let your food be your medicine."

As with other forms of yin and yang, the ideal diet is designed to achieve a balanced state of health. This means that we eat to remain receptive and sensitive to information and changes coming from our environment; this allows us to adapt to our environment. At the same time, we strive to remain strong and focused, so that we can influence our environment in the way that we wish. The goal of macrobiotics, therefore, is to create an optimal condition of health and mental clarity so that we can direct our energy efficiently toward the realization of our dreams.

Achieving a balance between yin and yang means eating a certain kind of diet.

In general, the yang, or contractive, foods are salt (the most contractive food available), red meat, eggs, chicken, and fish (going from most yang to lesser yang). Whole grains are seen as balanced on the yin-yang spectrum, though slightly on the yang side. Beans are slightly yin; root vegetables more yin than beans; leafy green vegetables more yin than roots; fruits more yin than vegetables; fruit juice more yin than fruit; and sugar more yin than juice. Drugs, which are said to have an "mind expanding" effect, are the most extreme yin, we can encounter, short of death.

Extreme yang foods will create a craving for extreme yin foods. Specifically, diets composed of salt, red meat, hard cheeses, eggs, and chicken, will have to include lots of fruit, sugar, and even alcohol in order for the person to feel balanced and satisfied.

In a temperate climate, a balanced diet is composed chiefly of whole grains, beans, a wide variety of fresh vegetables (including leafy greens, squashes, tubers, and roots), sea vegetables, fruit, and fish. (See dietary guidelines in Chapter 8.)

This diet is composed of foods that are at the center of the yin-yang spectrum. They do not represent extremes. Consequently, they will not cause extreme cravings for their opposites. One can feel satisfied with less extreme forms of yin and yang. The more yang your diet beomes, however, the more extreme kinds of yin you will need to feel at peace.

When cravings are reduced, it is much easier to eat simply and healthfully. What all of us are really striving for is balance and satisfaction. Imbalance is the source of hunger and cravings. The stronger the imbalance, the greater the hunger and craving. The way to treat extreme cravings is to restore and reduce the extremes in the diet. This will enable us to create balance with extreme-producing foods, such as meat, eggs, and chicken, all of which cause us to crave greater quantities of sugar and other extreme yin foods.

When you eat a balanced diet for awhile, your body becomes free of a lot of excess fat and cholesterol, and consequently you grow increasingly sensitive to your own health and condition. You naturally become more flexible and better able to adapt to changes in your environment. Also, you feel the effects of extreme foods, such as sugar, much more rapidly than you would have felt them in the past. Small deviations in your diet become obvious.

In macrobiotics, cooking is taken very seriously. Initially, that is often a challenging task; more time is needed to learn to prepare the foods and for awhile the cooking is more demanding than, say, tossing a potpie in the microwave.

However, as the saying goes, you get what you pay for—especially when it comes to the amount of time and energy you have invested in your health. By taking the time to prepare foods that support and encourage your health, you gain the luxury of forgetting about your body when you are working and playing. You have optimal amounts of energy; you have fewer days when you are sick and miserable; you look good with less effort;

you sleep soundly and wake up refreshed. You enjoy the freedom from drugs, headaches, body aches, and frequent attacks of the flu. You are no longer worn down; you look younger and feel younger. The little extra time you put into your cooking pays off in a multitude of ways, which usually save you time in the long run.

The key to remaining on the diet is to give yourself the time to learn to prepare the macrobiotic foods, and enjoy them. Your taste buds need time to adjust to a diet low in fat, cholesterol, salt, sugar, and artificial additives. Before long, you will wonder how you ever ate any other way.

Guidelines for Lowering Cholesterol Level and Reversing Atherosclerosis

1. *Avoid Red Meat.*   Most red meats are high in fat and cholesterol and, as a food group, are entirely unnecessary for health. As we saw in the previous chapter, many red meats contain more than half of their calories in fat. Ground beef, for example, contains, as much as 64 percent of its total calories in fat; stewing beef, 71 percent; rump roast, 71 percent; sirloin steak, lean with the fat still present, contains 75 percent; T-bone steak, lean with fat, 82 percent.

Red meat has numerous other drawbacks, as well. Most American livestock are fed antibiotics and hormones. The antibiotics are given as so-called *preventives* to ward off illnesses and cut down on loss of animals. Those antibiotics have given rise to resistant strains of bacteria, including salmonella, which is responsible for food poisoning. Consequently, an increasing number of resistant strains of viruses and bacterias are turning up which defy medical treatment.

Antibiotics have a widespread and deleterious effect on the health of humans. They destroy friendly intestinal flora, which are essential to proper digestion. By destroying these friendly bacteria, antibiotics encourage the growth of disease-promoting bacteria, such as candida albicans, or common yeast, which causes candidiasis.

Antibiotics also weaken immune response. Studies have shown

that by taking the place of the human immune function, antibiotics weaken our ability to ward off illnesses, and make us more dependent upon these drugs.

Livestock is also treated with hormones.

According to *The New York Times* (January 1, 1989), "Cattlemen use the hormones to speed the fattening process in steers and heifers during the 120 days before slaughter. A single $1 hormone pellet implanted in the animal's ear can save $20 in fattening costs and cut the feeding period by 18 days, increasing the number of animals that can be fattened at a feed lot each year." The hormones "desex" the animals. They become more calm, which allows more of them to be penned together in a confined area.

Seventy to 90 percent of all cattle in the United States are fed hormones. Chicken and pork are also routinely fed hormones, as well.

Residues of these hormones are present in the red meat people eat.

The entire European Community has banned hormone-treated beef from their markets. Despite pressure from the United States government, Europe has steadfastly refused to accept American-produced beef.

No one knows what the short- or long-term effects of such hormones are on human biology. The human hormonal balance is incredibly delicate. As we will see in Chapter 5, fat alone adversely changes hormonal balance and assists in the production of cancer cells.

Red meat is difficult to digest. Most of us cannot masticate a piece of red meat; consequently, it goes down our esophagus as a sinuous wad, a whole, indigestible mass that has a good chance of remaining within our intestinal tract for years. Red meat contributes to a variety of intestinal problems, including constipation, diverticulosis (pockets within the intestinal tract), and common cancers, including cancer of the colon, prostate, and breast.

For all of these reasons, red meats are unhealthful and unnecessary. We recommend you avoid it.

2. *Avoid Dairy Foods.* All whole milk products are high in
fat, and some are exceedingly high in fat. A cup of whole milk
contains 47 percent of its total calories in saturated fat. Whole
milk yogurt contains 48 percent of its total calories in fat; ice
cream, light, 48 percent; ice cream, rich, 64 percent and higher;
cheddar cheese, 71 percent; cream cheese, 90 percent.

The dependence upon milk and milk products is having
enormous consequences in the West. Like red meats and chicken,
milk also contains antibiotics and hormones. In April of 1985,
milk had to be taken off the shelves in Illinois because of a
widespread outbreak of salmonella poisoning. More than 2,000
cases were reported in five Midwestern states as a result of milk
tainted with salmonella, which is resistant to antibiotics. That
resistance was created because the animals were fed antibiotics,
causing the rise of resistant bacteria to manifest in the guts of
the animals. The resistant bacteria was then passed on in animal's milk, causing widespread food poisoning. Salmonella is
contagious, causing secondary infection once it is loose. Health
officials estimated that another 10,000 cases of food poisoning
would occur as a result of secondary infection.

The human body has trouble dealing with cow's milk, however. In addition to the fat, milk products contain lactose, the
sugar found in milk.

Milk is not consumed by most of the world's population after
weaning, usually by the age of two. Much of the world population is lactose intolerant, meaning that these people have lost
the enzyme lactase, which is necessary to digest the sugar found
in milk, lactose.

For these people, milk is a food of infancy and that giving up
milk is part of the normal process of maturation.

Those who continue to eat milk products—even those who are
not lactose intolerant—have trouble dealing with its side effects.
A study done by Harvard University scientists discovered that
the consumption of milk—or more specifically the consumption
of lactose—is a leading risk factor in the onset of ovarian cancer.
The Harvard research, which was published in *Lancet* on July 8,
1989, found that women with ovarian cancer have a lower than

normal level of transferase, an enzyme involved in the metabolism of dairy products. This enzyme assists in the digestion of lactose. The more lactose one consumes, the lower one's blood levels are of transferase. The researchers speculated that women with low levels of transferase who eat milk products—especially cottage cheese and yogurt—have three times the risk of contracting ovarian cancer.

Put simply, milk is not a food designed for human consumption. It was meant for baby cows. Our dependence upon milk and milk products has given rise to an endless array of health problems.

If you find it exceedingly difficult to give up milk entirely, then drink skim milk and eat skim milk products. At the same time, try to wean yourself of dairy foods.

3. *Avoid Eggs.*   One egg contains 250 milligrams of cholesterol, while 64 percent of its total calories come from fat. Enough said.

4. *Substitute Fish for Chicken.*   Chickens are fed antibiotics and hormones and live and die under such horrible conditions that to eat such a food is to invite disease. The dark meat and skin of chicken is high in fat—about 53 percent of its total calories come from fat. The light meat, without the skin, has about half that. If you are a lover of chicken, eat only the white meat and restrict yourself to chicken soup or small portions of white meat, approximately 3.5 ounces per serving. It is wise if you do not eat chicken any more than twice per month. If you can avoid it all together, so much the better.

Chicken is regarded as a yang food, which will cause you to be attracted to strong yin, such as excessive amounts of fruit and sugar. This will naturally cause more imbalance and have health effects.

Fish, especially white-meat fish, are low in fat and rich in protein. When you find yourself wanting animal food, eat fish. The flat fishes, such as flounder and soles, contain as little as 9 percent of their total calories in fat; Atlantic halibut contains 11 percent; scallops, 11 percent; and haddock, only 1 percent. Salmon is higher in polyunsaturated fats, which lower blood cholesterol. Salmon should be considered a treat or a break from the norm, however, because of its high fat content.

5. *Reduce Oils and Use Only High Quality Oils.* As we have said, oil is fat that is liquid at room temperature. Some oils, such as sesame, corn, safflower, and sunflower oils are polyunsaturated fats, which tend to lower blood cholesterol levels.

Most margarines, peanut, cottonseed, and soybean oils are monounsaturated fats, which tend to have a neutral effect on blood cholesterol levels. Olive oil is a monounsaturated fat that does appear to lower cholesterol level and blood pressure, according to numerous recent studies. Peanut, cottonseed, and soybean oil often turn up in highly processed foods, which combines them with ingredients that are unhealthful. Also, monounsaturated oils are often hydrogenated, causing them to be more saturated and thus more unhealthful.

Coconut, palm kernel, and palm oils contain saturated fats that raise blood cholesterol levels significantly, causing heart disease, cancer, and other illnesses.

Even polyunsaturated oils can cause illness. Studies have shown that polyunsaturated fats are also linked to cancer. Both poly- and monounsaturated fats become unstable and rancid, which cause free radical formation, which scientists now believe is the basis for tumor growth and atherosclerosis. Poly- and monounsaturated oils do raise blood fats and cause the rouleaux formation, which prevents blood and oxygen from getting to cells.

We recommend that oil be held to a minimum. Steam leafy greens and other vegetables and boil tubers and round vegetables. Use vegetables in soups. Sauté only occasionally: twice a week is a healthful rule of thumb. When you use oil, choose sesame oil and corn oil first, which are highly stable oils, meaning that they do not become rancid easily and form free radicals. Olive oil can be used occasionally (spring and summer are the most appropriate times) on salads and vegetables.

Reduce or avoid nut butters, such as peanut butter, tahini, and sesame butter. These nut butters are loaded with fat.

6. *Avoid Decaffeinated Coffee.* Coffee, in all its forms, is unhealthful. It causes a wide variety of symptoms, including increased heart and respiratory rates and elevated blood pressure. Studies have shown that coffee is implicated in the onset of heart disease and, when coupled with a diet high in fat, prostate cancer. In November 1989, Stanford University scientists reported that decaffeinated coffee significantly raised blood cholesterol levels, as much as 7 percent, and raised the chances of decaf drinkers suffering a heart attack some 12 to 14 percent. Decaf drinkers, the researchers found, experienced a rise of 9 mg/dl over non-decaf drinkers, including those who drank regular coffee. This elevation of cholesterol was due to the rise in LDL as a result of the decaffeinated coffee consumption.

7. *Avoid Refined White Sugar.* Sugar raises triglycerides which will elevate blood cholesterol levels somewhat. Sugar has many other unhealthful side effects. It causes hypoglycemia, explained in the next chapter, and weakens immune response, explained in Chapter 5.

8. *Adopt the Macrobiotic Dietary Guidelines.* As we have been saying all along, the macrobiotic diet is composed of whole grains, fresh vegetables, beans, sea vegetables, fruit, fish (if desired), and a wide assortment of condiments and soups. These foods are low in fat and cholesterol and rich in essential nutrients that promote health and vitality. The diet lowers blood cholesterol and can be instrumental in reversing atherosclerosis. The macrobiotic diet is fully explained in Chapter 8.

Chapter 4
Curing Overweight and Obesity and Achieving Optimal Weight

Can I lose weight and control my weight on the macrobiotic diet?

Like Lew Ross, Lynda Shoup suffered from a variety of illnesses, including obesity. In 1980, at the age of nineteen, Lynda weighed more than 200 pounds and stood only five feet two inches.

"You stop reading the scale after you reach 200 pounds," Lynda recalled. "You either adjust the dial on the scale so it won't give you an accurate reading, or you stop looking at all."

In addition to being overweight, Lynda suffered from severe asthma, food allergies, hypoglycemia, kidney stones, and had chronic bouts of lung disorders, especially pneumonia.

In 1985, she left her hometown of Torrington, Connecticut, and went to live in Tokyo, Japan. In 1986, she was introduced to acupuncture and then to macrobiotics. Lynda went to the acupuncturist for the kidney stones, but he informed her that if she did not change her diet, the kidney stones would continue to plague her. The acupuncturist said that Lynda's daily food was creating the stones, and that acupuncture could only provide symptomatic relief. He recommended that Lynda see an American macrobiotic teacher living in Tokyo, whose name was Phillip Jannetta. Jannetta put Lynda Shoup on a diet consisting mainly of whole grains, beans, fresh vegetables, sea vegetables, fermented foods, fruit, and natural sweeteners. The diet was low in fat and cholesterol, refined sugars, and artificial ingredients. Yet, it was rich in nutrients and highly satisfying to her taste.

For the next several months, Lynda dropped most of her excess weight, as well as her kidney stones, asthma, food allergies, and hypoglycemia.

By the end of 1986, Lynda Shoup weighed 138, "and still dropping," she says. Her weight has not come back since beginning macrobiotics. Nor have the other health problems she suffered from for so long.

Nancy Nickerson weighed a titanic 460 pounds in 1986. At five feet six inches tall, she fell into the catagory of "morbidly obese." She was thirty years old and everything she put in her mouth seemed to add several times its weight in body fat. That year, Nancy had decided to have her jaws wired shut, which would prevent her from eating anything but liquid foods. That seemed like her only hope of controlling her weight. She was about to go ahead with that decision when her grandmother died.

At the funeral, someone suggested to Nancy that she adopt a macrobiotic diet. The person also recommended someone who could cook all of Nancy's meals for her. Nancy was game. What did she have to lose? It seemed better than getting her jaw wired closed.

Her cook was not very adept at macrobiotic preparation, but that did not stop Nancy from losing 200 pounds in the first 13 months of her practice. Following that initial loss of weight, Nancy gradually lost another 100 pounds, and eventually dropped to a size "10–11" dress, where she has remained ever since.

Her blood cholesterol level went from 201 mg/dl to 125 mg/dl, where it has remained for the last four years.

According to the National Center for Health Statistics, 34 million American adults are overweight. Slightly more women suffer from overweight than do men; 27.1 percent of women exceed the ideal weight for their height, and 24.2 percent of men. The National Center for Health Statistics classifies overweight as 20 percent over the ideal weight for one's height. Many authorities say that such a weight can be considered obese.

A study done by the University of Michigan showed that women between the ages of eighteen to thirty-four are gaining weight more rapidly than men in that age group. The study showed that during the past several decades, the number of young women who now fall into the overweight category has been growing faster than the number of men who can be considered overweight. This is ironic because many sociologists believe that women are under greater pressure to be thin than men are under.

Women are not the only group gaining weight rapidly, however. Twenty percent of all children and adolescents are significantly overweight or obese. Scientists maintain that the reasons for this growing population of overweight children and adults is a culture addicted to fast foods, television, and a generally sedentary way of life.

Obesity is a risk factor in the onset of virtually every serious degenerative disease, including heart disease, cancer, high blood pressure, and diabetes. In other words, overweight is not the only problem facing the obese person. Also, excess weight, as we will see shortly in this chapter, reduces life expectancy all by itself. When you add the other illnesses that occur as a result of overweight, you have a person facing an extremely high risk of premature illness and death.

Conversely, the daily consumption of fewer calories and the condition of being slightly underweight is related to an incredible array of health benefits, including a stronger immune function, resistance to cancer, heart disease, diabetes, environmental pollutants, and the aging process. The benefits of eating foods lower in calories cannot be overestimated. Scientists believe that by eating fewer calories each day, people can extend their lives by as much as 50 percent.

"The outcome of caloric restriction is spectacular," Dr. Richard Weindruch, a gerontologist at the National Institute of Aging told *The New York Times* (April 17, 1990). "Gerontologists have tried many things to extend life span, but this is the only one that consistently works in the lab."

A diet low in calories actually protects the genes and body from environmental insults, while on the macroscopic level it serves to protect and enhance the strength and function of every organ. A low calorie diet has been shown to suppress the growth of tumors in laboratory animals.

"Right now, the maximum human life span is about 110 years, and only a few people live to that age," said Dr. Roy L. Walford, a professor of pathology at the University of California at Los Angeles (UCLA) School of Medicine. "But if what is true for other species is true for man, then with a sufficiently vigorous caloric restriction, the maximum life span could be extended to about 170."

The average daily calorie intake in the United States is about 2,500 calories per day. Scientists say that the life enhancing properties of a low calorie diet begin to take effect on a diet of 1,500 to 2,000 calories a day. Scientists point out that this number of calories is easily achieved on a diet composed chiefly of whole grains and vegetables, foods considered the healthiest by nutritionists.

How is weight loss accomplished on the macrobiotic diet?

Weight gain or weight loss occur according to a simple principle. Weight is gained when we eat more calories than we burn in activity. Weight is lost when we burn more calories than we take in. The whole trick to losing weight, therefore, is to take in fewer calories than we burn everyday. That causes us to burn our stored energy, which exists in the form of body fat. Unfortunately, most people read this and immediately say to themselves: "That means that I have to go hungry through most of the day." But that is not the case on the macrobiotic diet. You can eat until you are satisfied and you will still lose weight, as long as you adhere to the basic dietary principles. You will lose weight even faster if you follow some simple lifestyle guidelines, which we will outline below.

As for the diet, there are two foods that must be reduced or avoided if you are going to lose weight. Those foods are fat and refined sugar. Notice that we did not say that you must avoid a sweet flavor; there are lots of ways to enjoy a sweet dessert and avoid sugar. While you abstain from fat and sugar, you must increase whole grains, fresh vegetables, and beans. In short, you must increase complex carbohydrates.

Let us begin by looking at why the macrobiotic diet causes weight loss, and specifically how avoiding fat and sugar causes weight loss.

Fat

One way scientists determine the value of a specific food is to measure how many calories are present in the food itself. Calories are used to measure the potential energy of a food. Something with no calories will provide no energy. But something with a lot of calories will provide a lot of potential energy. It is up to you to use all that potential energy in your daily activities. Many foods provide more calories than we can burn. The calories that are not used will be converted to body fat, which, of course, causes weight gain.

You must keep in mind that food fats are calorically dense. That means that a teaspoon of fat will have many more calories than, say, a teaspoon of carbohydrates—about twice as many, in fact. For every gram of carbohydrate or protein, you get about four calories; for every gram of fat, you get about nine calories. You can eat the same volume of carbohydrates as fat, but you get twice the calories when you eat fatty foods.

While fats are rich in calories, they are empty of nutrients. Fats make up between 40 and 50 percent of the total calories of the typical American diet. That means that a great percentage of food we take in is empty of nutrients, which places increased demands on the remainder of our diets to provide the nutrition our body needs.

Therefore, the first and most important step to losing weight is to avoid foods that are rich in fat. These foods are red meat, dairy products, and eggs. If you want to lose weight, but insist on eating these foods, you will have to fast and exercise a great deal. The reason? When you eat fatty foods, you must go through periods of abstinence and increased exercise to burn excess calories. Still, it is unlikely that you will be able to burn off all the calories present in a fatty meal, which means you will gain weight.

If you sit down to a meal of steak, potatoes with sour cream, vegetables glazed in butter, salad drenched in French dressing, and chocolate mousse for dessert, you will have to decide whether to go out and chop wood for about four weeks—or do some equally demanding exercise—or watch yourself put on more body fat, and more pounds. That is the only choice you have. The reason is simple: you have just taken in several thousand calories, which have to be burned as fuel or converted to body fat. In other words, it is very hard to lose weight and stay on the typical American diet.

Fortunately, there is another way. You can change the basic composition of your diet. You can avoid high calorie foods, and eat whole grains, vegetables, beans, small amounts of fish, and more natural sweeteners.

You can have a full course meal that includes everything from soup to dessert, and lose weight. You can also stop counting calories. Counting calories does not work anyway—all it does is to instill guilt. The way we can become nutritionally and sensorially satisfied is to adopt the macrobiotic diet.

The macrobiotic diet is very low in fat; only 10 to 15 percent of its total calories come from fat. Virtually all the foods that make up the diet are low in fat and cholesterol.

The primary foods in the macrobiotic diet are whole grains, fresh vegetables, beans, sea vegetables, fruit, natural sweeteners, fish, and a variety of condiments and soups. Once you learn how to prepare these foods, you will recognize that there is far more variety in the macrobiotic diet than there is in the standard American diet. There is also far more varied flavors and textures. What is more, you can be happy eating this way, and fully satisfied, while you watch yourself lose weight. This is a well-documented fact.

At Brigham Young University, in Provo, Utah, scientists took obese women and placed them on a diet rich in complex carbohydrates from grains and vegetables and low in fat. The scientists did not restrict the women from eating as much as they wanted—none of the participants ever had to fast; neither were they encouraged to exercise. Yet, they still lost weight.

Obese "people can still lose weight without feeling starved," said A. Garth Fisher, Ph.D., professor of physical education at Brigham Young University, who was among the researchers conducting the study. "Changing diet composition in favor of a higher carbohydrate-to-fat ration without conscious restriction of calories from exercise results in a significant decrease in weight." The study was published in the January 1989 issue of *The American Journal of Clinical Nutrition*.

In addition to being low in fat, the macrobiotic diet is made up of foods that are rich in nutrition and fiber.

Whole foods are nutritionally balanced; that is, they are composed of varying amounts of the full complement of nutrients nature invested in them. Whole grain brown rice, for example, contains complex carbohydrates, protein, minerals, vitamins, fat, and fiber. Brown rice addresses every need of the body— carbohydrates for energy; protein for cell replacement and repair; minerals and vitamins for cell metabolism and immune strength; small amounts of fat for energy reserves; and fiber to assist digestion and elimination. The same is true of whole grains; all whole vegetables; and all whole beans. We are not saying that anyone should eat only whole grains; the macrobiotic diet is rich in variety and no one food should be eaten to the exclusion of all others on the diet. What we are saying is that the body needs a balance of nutrients that can only be found in whole, unrefined foods.

There is another advantage to whole foods that is important to people who want to lose weight.

Whole foods have bulk, most of which is fiber and water. This bulk fills the stomach and gives the feeling of being sated. As Nathan Pritikin points out in his book, *The Pritikin Permanent Weight-Loss Manual*, the stomach contains about four cups of volume. In order to feel satisfied, the stomach needs to have the experience of being full. You can load the stomach with four cups of fat and protein, or four cups of natural whole foods, such as whole grains, vegetables, beans, and fruit. The net effect will be that if the stomach is filled with fat and protein, you are going to gain weight—fast! If it is filled with whole grains and vegetables, you are going to lose weight.

In both cases, the stomach will be full, but even the experience of fullness will be different. When you eat a heavy meal of red meat, sauces, and various foods with dairy and eggs in them, the feeling of fullness you get is almost oppressive. The stomach must expand beyond comfortable proportions; it is so heavily weighed down by such a meal that you begin to feel sleepy. The reason you want to sleep is because your body's energy must be diverted to the stomach and intestines in order to perform the Herculean task of digesting this type of food. The only way such a feat can be performed is if you rest while your stomach and intestines deal with your meal. In all likelihood, there will be immediate symptoms of distress: stomach cramps, heartburn, acidic stomach, or intestinal discomfort.

However, a meal that is composed of grains and vegetables, or fish and vegetables, is lighter, rich in fiber, and much easier to digest. Consequently, the demands on your digestive tract are not nearly as great. You do not feel sleepy after such a meal; nor do you feel the need for Pepto Bismal, or Tums, or Alka Seltzer. This means that the body can handle such a meal easily and efficiently, while you go about doing whatever you want to do when the meal is concluded.

Sugar

Another important factor in losing weight is the avoidance of sugar in your daily diet. Like fat, sugar is a source of "empty" calories. This means that you get lots of calories from sugar, but no nutrition. This leads to both weight gain and fluctuating blood sugar levels, called *hypoglycemia*. (As we will see in Chapter 5, sugar also has a detrimental effect on the immune system.) Let us deal with the question of weight gain first.

Sugar is produced by extracting simple carbohydrates from sugar cane or sugar beets. A whole sugar beet weighs, on the average, about two pounds and contains a full complement of nutrients—complex carbohydrates, minerals, vitamins, protein, and fiber. A whole sugar beet provides about 500 calories, but it is unlikely that you would sit down and eat a whole, two-pound sugar beet, even if you loved sugar beets. When a sugar

beet is reduced to refined white sugar, however, all the nutrients
are thrown away, except the carbohydrates, which are converted
to simple carbohydrates. Now that two-pound sugar beet is
reduced to four-and-a-half ounces of refined sugar, which also
contains 500 calories. It is very easy for people to eat four-and-
a-half ounces of sugar. If you compare the calories found in
that two-pound sugar beet—500—to the calories found in two
pounds of refined sugar—3,500—you begin to recognize how
important it is to avoid sugar and all refined foods.

Sugar, Weight Gain, and Behavior

Refined white sugar enters your bloodstream the minute you
put a food containing sugar in your mouth. This immediately
elevates the glucose levels in your blood and causes you to feel
an initial rush of energy. The blood sugar is quickly burned as
fuel or converted to fat. Once it is burned or stored, the sugar
levels in your blood drop precipitously, falling below fasting
levels. This causes you to feel lethargic, fatigued, and drained of
energy. A variety of emotional reactions often occur, such as
depression, irritability, anger, and anxiety. Many people feel an
unexplained nervous tension, as well. This weakened state,
typically referred to as hypoglycemia, affects millions of people.
It is so common that certain candy bar companies take advantage
of it by suggesting that when you feel these symptoms you should
have a candy bar for a "pick-me-up." The candy bar provides
another rush of energy, but creates the same downward spiral
to occur all over again, keeping your energy levels and moods
on a perpetual roller coaster ride. The sense of weakness, loss of
control, and fluctuating energy combine to affect many people
deeply, creating enormous insecurities.

In this way, sugar is addictive. It creates an initial energy rush,
but soon deprives a person of both energy and emotional stability.
Consequently, you need another burst of sugar to restore your
energy to its previous level, but that new round of sugar is
quickly burned, and you are left feeling depleted and craving
sugar all over again.

But it goes even deeper than that. Sugar is a fuel for cells. In addition to fuel, cells need vitamins and minerals to carry on metabolism. When you eat a food that is rich in sugar, or fuel, cells are set in motion, but still need nutrients to carry on their metabolic activities. If the food is empty of nutrients, however, the cells must draw these nutrients from some other place, such as teeth, bones, and other tissues, if they are to perform their tasks. In other words, the consumption of sugar results in a net loss of nutrients and a general weakening of the body.

Dr. Derrick Lonsdale at the Cleveland Clinic found that adolescents who ate a diet rich in simple sugars suffered from low thiamine levels and the early signs of beriberi. Those symptoms included irritability, mood swings, fatigue, depression, insomnia, and chest and abdominal pains. Thiamine is required by the body to utilize sugar. As sugar intake is increased, thiamine levels decrease. When Lonsdale added more thiamine to the children's diet, including the addition of whole grains and vegetables which are rich in thiamine, their symptoms disappeared.

Food dramatically affects the way we feel. Indeed, it immediately affects brain chemistry.

Writing in the December 1979 issue of *Nutrition Action*, a publication of the Center for Science in the Public Interest, Dr. John Fernstrom stated that, "It is becoming increasingly clear that brain chemistry and function can be influenced by a single meal." Fernstrom, a research scientist at the Massachusetts Institute of Technology, pointed out that, "in well-nourished individuals consuming normal amounts of food, short-term changes in food composition can rapidly affect brain function."

Research at MIT has demonstrated that sugar causes the blood to be flooded with an amino acid called *tryptophan*, which is converted in the brain to a neurotransmitter called *serotonin*. Elevated levels of serotonin cause a heightened sense of well-being, better sleep, and improved mood. But MIT researchers have found that obese people use sugar as a drug to keep themselves from feeling depressed and anxious. When the sugar-induced serotonin wears off, these people feel a rise in anxiety and depression, which is alleviated by a new round of sugar.

Dr. Richard Wurtman, who along with his wife, Dr. Judith Wurtman, conducted the study at MIT, stated: "I think they [the obese people] were using food as a drug."

Of course, this craving for sugars is addictive and causes additional weight gain. It is a never-ending cycle that keeps the overweight person overweight and depressed.

The effects of complex carbohydrates, found in whole grains, vegetables, beans, and fruit, are far different than that found in simple sugars. Complex carbohydrates are made up of long chains of carbohydrate molecules that must be broken down in the intestines to be made available to the bloodstream as sugar. Instead of overloading the blood with a sudden quantity of sugar, complex carbohydrates are broken down inside the intestines in a steady and methodical fashion, providing steady and consistent energy. The effect is that you have long-term energy and endurance between breakfast and lunch, and then between lunch and supper. Complex carbohydrates free us from the roller coaster ride of energy and lethargy that simple sugars cause.

Complex carbohydrates also cause the brain to secrete more serotonin, which provides a sense of well-being and safety. One feels emotionally "centered" and balanced on a diet that is rich in complex carbohydrates.

Additionally, complex carbohydrates usually come from whole foods, which provide an abundance of other nutrients, such as protein, minerals, vitamins, and fiber. The body is getting what it needs to support itself. Refined foods, on the other hand, are stripped of much of their nutrition, which causes the body to leach minerals and vitamins from tissues in order to meet its nutritional needs.

One nutrient that is essential, especially for people who want to lose weight, is fiber. Fiber, which is the undigestible portion of grains, vegetables, and fruit, enhances our ability to eliminate waste. Without fiber, we are more likely to suffer from constipation and related bowel problems. Undigested matter remains in the intestinal tract longer, which causes toxins to enter the bloodstream and causes illnesses elsewhere in the body. One study, reported in the British medical journal, *Lancet* (2, 1981: 1203), showed that women who suffer from chronic constipation are far more likely to suffer from breast disease, including malignant tumors, than those who have at least one bowel movement per day.

Chronic intestinal problems can lead to diverticulosis, an illness characterized by pockets forming in the intestinal tract, where undigested matter remains for long periods of time. This adds weight, prevents efficient elimination, and weakens our ability to absorb nutrients.

When the small intestine is coated with fat, nutrient absorption is diminished, often causing us to desire more food to meet our nutrient needs. This, of course, increases caloric intake and quickly adds weight.

The Importance of Chewing

Mahatma Gandhi said "Drink your food and eat your soup," and better advice was never given.

Nothing enhances digestion, nor increases our ability to absorb nutrients, better than chewing. The importance of chewing cannot be overstated. The more we chew, the more we break up food particles, making them easier to assimilate in the small intestine. With excellent chewing, we place less stress on our stomach and small intestine to deal with food bulk, and enhance our ability to eliminate.

Chewing causes the secretion of saliva, which exposes our food to greater quantities of digestive enzymes, which prepare the food for digestion and assimilation. Saliva also causes the food to be alkalized, which makes it harmonious with the stomach's acidic environment. If we fail to chew, our food enters the stomach in a more acidic state, which can cause heartburn, ulcers, and other digestive disorders.

Not surprisingly, the more you chew your food, the less food you need to feel satisfied. That is, the more you chew, the easier it is to feel full and satisfied. Of course, this only stands to reason: the more you chew, the easier it is for your body to extract the nutrients it needs from the food.

At the Kushi Institute in Becket, Massachusetts, Michio Kushi teaches his students to chew every mouthful 150 times. Students uniformly report that after a day or so of chewing this way, their cravings for foods outside the diet, as well as their need for larger quantities of food, greatly diminishes. Students can eat more simply and far less.

You should chew your food at least fifty to seventy times per mouthful. Not only will this dramatically affect your eating habits and health, but it will also change the extent to which you are able to taste your food. As an experiment, chew a mouthful of grain, say brown rice, in your normal fashion. Then chew the next mouthful 100 times and see the difference in taste. You will find your brown rice is much sweeter and tastier when you chew it 100 times per mouthful. You will also need less food to feel full and satisfied. Chewing is one of the fundamental keys to good health, and especially to controlling weight. Do not underestimate this tool. If you want to control your appetite effortlessly, chew your food copiously—at least fifty to seventy times per mouthful—and watch the pounds effortlessly slip away.

Yin and Yang, Food Cravings, and Hunger

As we explained in the previous chapter, yin and yang are complementary opposites that are always attracting each other. Yin attracts yang and yang attracts yin.

The attraction of yin and yang is the underlying reason for all hunger, cravings, and attractions. No matter what you crave —some type of food or love—your hunger is an imbalanced state. You feel empty or lacking in some way. This can be seen as yang, or a contracted state. In hunger, the stomach is more contracted; the cells are craving nutrition; and the desire to "fill up," or expand .. at its peak.

Food causes a more yin state, at least initially. The stomach expands; one feels sated and more restful; and in general, one feels more balanced after a meal (though it often depends on the meal, and the degree of hunger one experienced prior to the meal).

If you eat an excess of salt, which is an extreme form of yang, you will crave sweet foods, or some other form of strong yin, such as alcohol. If you eat sugar and drink alcohol, you will naturally crave strong yang foods, such as meat, eggs, and salt. It goes both ways, yin and yang are always attempting to make balance and harmony. A diet composed of meat and sugar does create a degree of balance, but these foods have side effects. Meat is rich in fat and cholesterol; cattle, pigs, chickens, and other livestock are fed antibiotics, and steroids, which you ingest when you eat these foods. This diet, though it creates a degree of balance, is a formula for sickness.

If you eat less extreme yang foods—fish for example—you will need smaller and less severe yin foods to make balance with the yang aspects of your diet. The macrobiotic diet is composed of foods that are less extreme forms of yin and yang—fish, grains, vegetables, and fruit. Consequently, you will feel satisfied with less extreme forms of yin and yang. You will not crave strong yin or yang because both these archetypal forces are always making balance.

The macrobiotic diet is designed to create a more harmonious state within. As you get to know the foods on the diet and become more adept at cooking them, your cravings will become less intense and you will find yourself far more satisfied than ever before.

Guidelines for Losing Weight

1. Eat only when you are truly hungry.
2. Make whole foods, especially whole grains, the center of your diet.
3. Vary your foods widely. Eat a variety of whole grains, and a wide variety of vegetables, beans, sea vegetables, and fruit.
4. Chew every mouthful of food at least 50 times, preferably 75 to 100 times. Chewing will provide you with a maximum sense of satiation on a minimum of food. The more you chew, the less you need to eat; at the same time, the more you chew, the less hunger you will feel.

5. Do not overeat. Ideally, we should eat to the point of being 80 percent full. This will be considerably easier the more you chew your food. The more you chew, the more you will feel full and satisfied on less.

6. Avoid dietary fat, especially saturated fat, and oily foods, which are loaded with excess calories. Eat fish before poultry and poultry before red meat. When you eat poultry, avoid the dark meat and the skin, both of which are high in fat.

7. Avoid sugar and refined foods. When you crave a sweet taste, eat foods that are sweetened with less refined sweeteners, such as yinnie rice syrup, barley malt, or apple juice. Also, make sure your desserts include a whole grain, such as whole wheat or brown rice, so that the dessert will include more nutrition and greater fiber.

8. Do not eat at least three hours before retiring to bed each night. This will give your body time to digest your food. It will also help you to get a better night's sleep, during which much healing takes place.

9. Take a brisk walk everyday, weather permitting. Walking is the ideal exercise; it burns calories and reduces stress. It gives you time to think clearly and restore perspective to your life. (See Chapter 7 on exercise.) Make your walk at least thirty minutes long.

10. Be active. Avoid watching television or spending too much time sitting. Fill your day with more of the things you need to do and want to do. In other words, get as much done each day as possible.

11. Avoid extremes in yin and yang. Make the majority of your foods balanced at the center of the yin-yang spectrum. These foods include whole grains, fresh vegetables (especially leafy greens and roots), beans, sea vegetables, fish, and fruit.

12. Follow the 30 Days Program outlined in Chapter 9.

Chapter 5

Diet, Cancer, Adult-onset Diabetes: Diet as Cause and Treatment

You said in Chapter 1 that heart disease, cancer, and other illnesses are actually one disease. How are these illnesses related?

Before we launch into our discussion, let us have a look at the facts, namely those emerging from the largest and most comprehensive study of dietary habits and disease patterns ever done. The research, conducted by Cornell University scientists, examined the diets and disease rates of 6,500 Chinese and was called the "Grand Prix" of epidemiology research by *The New York Times*.

The study of Chinese dietary patterns and disease rates revealed that the Chinese diet, which consists overwhelmingly of whole grains and vegetables and very small amounts of animal foods, protects against virtually all the common degenerative diseases, including heart disease, cancer, osteoporosis, diabetes, and high blood pressure.

The Chinese eat 20 percent more calories than Americans do, but obesity is rare among Chinese. The reason for the difference: Chinese eat only a third as much fat as Americans and twice the complex carbohydrates from grains and vegetables. Complex carbohydrate foods are easily burned as fuel or consumed by the body to produce heat. In other words, they are not readily converted into fat.

Not only do the Chinese consume less fat, but also lower levels of protein and dramatically smaller amounts of animal protein. The Chinese eat a third less protein overall than Americans. Meanwhile, only 7 percent of their protein comes from animal foods, while 70 percent of the American protein comes from animal sources. Animal proteins have been linked to a number of degenerative diseases, including cancer and osteoporosis.

Chinese rates of cancer are low, the result of their low fat and low cholesterol intake. Breast and reproductive cancers are rare in China. Since early menarche has been linked to the consumption of animal foods, fat, and high calorie intake, Chinese women, not surprisingly, begin menstruation three to six years later than Americans.

Most Chinese do not consume dairy products, yet osteoporosis is rare in China. Interestingly, the Chinese consume only half the calcium Americans do. They get their calcium almost exclusively from plant foods, such as leafy green vegetables (see Chapter 8 for plant sources of calcium).

The Chinese blood cholesterol levels are also uniformly low. They range from 88 mg/dl to 165 mg/dl, nearly half of what Americans average, which is from 155 mg/dl to 274 mg/dl.

And just as we have been saying throughout this book, blood cholesterol is a good indicator of illness. Chinese diets do differ somewhat between rich and poor. Also, there are some regional dietary differences. Where the fat and cholesterol consumption is higher, the disease rates are higher.

"So far we've seen that plasma cholesterol is a good predictor of the kinds of diseases people are going to get," said Dr. T. Colin Campbell, biochemist at Cornell and organizer of the study. "Those with higher cholesterol levels are prone to the diseases of affluence—cancer, heart disease, and diabetes," said Dr. Campbell.

After reviewing the evidence his researchers compiled—which had been published by Cornell in a 920 page book—Dr. Campbell summarized his thoughts this way:

"We're basically a vegetarian species and should be eating a wide variety of plant foods and minimizing our intake of animal foods."

Dr. Campbell went further:

"Usually, the first thing a country does in the course of economic development is to introduce a lot of livestock. Our data are showing that this is not a very smart move, and the

Chinese are listening. They're realizing that animal-based agriculture is not the way to go."

Many Forms of One Disease, with One Cause

The common forms of heart disease, cancer, adult-onset diabetes, high blood pressure, and many of the illnesses associated with aging all stem from our daily food. The illnesses that afflict tens of millions are really a single disease that, for lack of a better term, we can call food poisoning. The principle poison is fat. But there are other poisons in the diet—excess protein (especially animal protein), refined grains and sugar, and common additives, such as artificial colors, flavors, preservatives, and pesticides.

These foods and ingredients combine to poison the body and create symptom states which we refer to as specific illnesses, such as certain cancers, coronary heart disease, adult-onset diabetes, or osteoporosis. But each of these are really branches of one illness. How that disease manifests in individual people depends on the person's genetic strengths and weaknesses, his daily behavior patterns, and what kinds of foods have predominated in his diet.

In this chapter, we will look at some of the common degenerative illnesses that afflict people young and old and how they are related to our common eating patterns, especially to our intake of fat and cholesterol. In the next chapter, we will look at disorders associated with aging. Let us begin here with cancer.

Cancer

Cancer rates continue to climb at a frightening pace and more people are dying of cancer today than ever before. Approximately one million Americans are diagnosed with cancer each year and about 500,000 die annually from this dread disease.

The American Cancer Society and the National Cancer Institute would like you to believe that "we are winning the war on cancer." They juggle the numbers to create the illusion that fully half of all people who contract cancer are "cured," meaning that they are alive five years after diagnosis. That, unfortunately, is untrue.

The General Accounting Office (GAO), which assesses policy and governmental practices for the U.S. Congress, reported in 1987 that medical gains in treating cancer have been "overstated" and inflated by the National Cancer Institute, the leading cancer research center in the United States. The GAO stated that between 1950 and 1982 there has been little or no progress made in the treatment of the majority of the twelve most common tumors. The numbers of people reported "cured" of cancer are interpreted in such a way to make people believe that progress is being made rapidly, but this is not the case, GAO stated.

Early detection of cancer has improved somewhat, which often accounts for longer life span between diagnosis and death. However, the NCI has suggested that cancer therapies are responsible for this longer life span between diagnosis and death, and that progress is being made in the *treatment* of cancer. This, said the GAO, just is not true.

In the past few years, numerous articles have appeared—in such places as the vaunted *New England Journal of Medicine*—that have reinterpreted the statistics on cancer recoveries and offered a much gloomier picture. Despite the $80 billion spent each year on cancer research, two-out-of-three people with cancer will die within five years of diagnosis. That is the same number that were dying in 1950. The only difference is that more people are contracting cancer today than forty years ago. That increase is in real numbers, meaning that more people today die from cancer per 100,000 population than ever before.

Meanwhile, scientists carry on an enormous public relations effort to make it appear that the billions of dollars lavished on research is money well spent.

Clearly, another approach is needed.

That approach is prevention. And prevention begins by putting a stop to the poisons that are the source of the problem. But prevention is more than keeping people healthy. It is a kind of personal and social treatment. We are treating cancer by stopping it at its cause. Why we need to have cancer manifest at all is the question. Why wait until cancer is raging inside of us before we take steps against this illness? Why not treat the causes of the disease before they are able to gain too strong a grip on us? The methods of cancer prevention are well-established in the scientific literature. Indeed, such preventive measures as diet, exercise, the cessation of smoking, and the elimination of certain strong carcinogens from our immediate environment have been more thoroughly researched than many of the treatments being offered today, and proven to be more effective.

Let us have a look at some of that research and how we can use it to protect us against cancer.

Preventing Cancer with Diet

"The forms of cancer that appear to be dependent on nutrition as shown by epidemiological studies include: stomach, liver, breast, prostate, large intestine, small intestine, and colon," said former director of the National Cancer Institute, Dr. Gio Gori.

Dr. Ernst Wynder, medical director of the American Health Foundation and a leading expert on cancer stated that, "Breast cancer, the biggest killer of all cancers in women, has a geographical distribution similar to that of colon cancer and is also associated worldwide with the consumption of a high fat diet."

In 1979, the U.S. Surgeon General published *Healthy People: The U.S. Surgeon General's Report on Health Promotion and Disease Prevention*. Among the Surgeon General's findings was that the scientific evidence overwhelmingly demonstrated that the common cancers were associated with a high fat diet.

In 1982, the National Research Council published *Diet, Nutrition, and Cancer*, which stated that a "causal" relationship existed between the common cancers and a high fat diet.

The Surgeon General, the National Research Council, the U.S. Departments of Agriculture and Health and Human Services have all recommended that people reduce their fat and cholesterol intake in order to prevent cancer, heart disease, and other degenerative illnesses. These government and scientific agencies have urged people to eat more whole grains, fresh vegetables, fruit, and fish. The Surgeon General specifically stated that Americans should eat less red meat to protect themselves against disease.

The reason for these recommendations is that the scientific consensus urging dietary change is overwhelming.

Let us look at the common cancers and their origins to better understand the relationship between our eating habits and cancer.

Colon Cancer

Scientists have found that fat consumption and a lack of fiber from whole grains, vegetables, and fruit combine to create the perfect intestinal environment for colon cancer. A high fat diet causes an increase in the body's production of bile acids, which are used to help digest fat. The more fat in the diet, the more the body secretes bile into the intestinal tract. Together, the fat and bile deplete oxygen levels in the intestines and create the ideal conditions for anaerobic bacteria, which proliferate in oxygen-deprived conditions. These anaerobic bacteria convert bile acids into powerful carcinogens, which trigger the onset of malignancy.

The lack of fiber slows intestinal transit time—the amount of time it takes for waste to move through the intestinal tract and then be eliminated from the body. As intestinal transit time is delayed, the intestines are exposed to toxins that would otherwise be eliminated more rapidly. These toxins also add to the unhealthful conditions within the digestive tract.

According to the National Research Council (NRC), these conditions promote the transformation of cholic acid, a common constituent in the intestines, into a powerful carcinogen.

Dr. Denis Burkitt, who studied the diets and health of African tribes, discovered that, because of their high fiber diet, the African people have little or no incidence of intestinal cancer.

Other studies reported by the National Cancer Institute have shown that dietary fiber shrinks precancerous polyps in the intestinal tract. These polyps can become malignant. Fiber, found in whole grains and vegetables, was found to inhibit and even reverse the process by which a lesion in the colon becomes cancerous.

The NRC found that cholesterol in the bowel increases tumor growth. The more cholesterol, the more greater incidence of tumor development, the NRC noted. In *Diet, Nutrition, and Cancer*, the NRC reported that tumor growth increased dramatically in animal studies when their diets reached 20 percent total calories from fat. Most Americans get between 35 and 45 percent of their total calories from fat.

Breast Cancer

The rate of death from breast cancer is increasing at an alarming rate in the United States. Between 1979 and 1986, breast cancer rates in the United States rose 31 percent. In 1990, 150,000 new cases of breast cancer will be diagnosed, and if the present trend continues that number will increase significantly throughout the next decade.

Despite convincing evidence that had been building for decades, many scientists doubt the link between dietary fat and breast cancer. The National Cancer Institute decided to cancel two major studies examining the relationship between diet and breast cancer. The reason the studies were cancelled was that some scientists doubt the link between diet and breast disease, and argue that even if such a link exists, they still do not know the mechanisms by which fat would initiate malignancy in the breast. These scientists maintain that the cost of such studies—one of the breast cancer projects would have cost $130 million—was just too much to justify.

The cancellations of both studies aroused controversy and anger. Feminists argued that this was just another example of men deciding the fate of women's health. Activists called the decision to reject both studies a "travesty." One activist said, "For men, they spend."

The irony is that smaller research projects have long demonstrated a strong connection between fat intake and breast cancer. A January 1990 issue of the *Journal of the National Cancer*

Institute published a report demonstrating that women could cut their risk of breast cancer four to five times by eating a diet low in fat, especially saturated fat.

Dr. Barry Goldin of Tuft's University Medical School, one of the researchers who conducted the study, urged women to reduce their fat intake to 25 percent of their total calories.

A study published in August 1988 issue of the *Journal of the National Cancer Institute* demonstrated that dietary fat consumed one year prior to diagnosis of breast cancer may well affect the growth and spread of the disease. The study, conducted by Canadian researchers from Laval University in Quebec City, found that consumption of fat also predicted the severity of the disease. High intake of saturated fat correlated more frequently with cancerous involvement of the lymph nodes, a much more serious stage of the disease than when it is localized in the breast.

A February 1989 issue of the *Journal of the National Cancer Institute* reported a study demonstrating that women who consumed a high fat diet had two to three times the rate of breast cancer than women who ate a diet low in fat.

Interestingly, the researchers demonstrated that the foods that seemed to increase the risk of breast cancer the most were high fat dairy products, mostly whole milk and cheese.

According to Tuft's Barry Goldin, low fat diets reduce the body's production of estrogens. Lower levels of estrogens are associated with lower risk of breast cancer.

Fat has been shown to increase the hormone prolactin, which governs estrogen and milk production. Increased levels of estrogen have been shown to fuel the growth of cancer cells.

Fat accumulation in the intestinal tract increases anaerobic bacteria and the production of estrogens, which travel throughout the body via the bloodstream. These estrogens further enhance tumor development at specific cites, including the breast. Estrogens produced by anaerobic bacteria have been shown to adversely affect reproductive organs and create cysts, as well.

Higher levels of estrogen have been found in women with breast cancer and men with bowel and prostate cancer.

Some researchers now believe that a high fat diet initiates the disease process early in life and that consumption of a high fat diet during adulthood promotes the disease.

Female children who eat a high fat diet and women with cancer have been shown to have higher than normal levels of prolactin. Research has shown that high prolactin levels can adversely affect breast tissue and the endocrine system during childhood, predisposing young girls to breast disease later on.

In the March 1987 issue of the *American Journal of Clinical Nutrition*, scientists reported that dietary fat causes the accumulation of cytotoxins, or substances that injure cells, in the intestinal tract. These cytotoxins spread throughout the body via the blood and can cause cell aberrations in any number of places, including the breast and sexual organs.

Drs. Nicholas L. Petrakis and Eileen B. King of the University of California published a report in the British medical journal, *Lancet*, that found that women who had two or fewer bowel movements per week had four times the risk of breast disease—both benign and malignant—than women who had a daily bowel movement.

After taking samples of breast fluid from 5,000 women, the physicians found a direct correlation between the number of abnormal cells in the breast fluid with the frequency of bowel movements. Those women who suffered from chronic constipation contained more abnormal cells than those who had a daily bowel elimination.

Studies have long shown that people who eat meat have a greater number of mutagenic agents (substances that cause cell mutation) than those who abstain from meat and whose diets consist of a greater proportion of vegetables.

Other studies have shown that total caloric intake directly affects cancer rates, especially breast cancer rates. Women who consume fewer calories show a lower level of breast cancer.

Finally, studies have shown that alcohol consumption is a major risk factor of breast cancer. Studies have shown that as few as three drinks per week place a woman at greater risk of breast cancer.

Prostate Cancer

Prostate cancer is also a fat- and hormone-related illness, as well. Studies have shown that prostate cancer was unheard of in Japan prior to 1950, but increased dramatically as meat and fat consumption increased in that country, according to the NRC. Laboratory studies have demonstrated consistently that prostate cancer is directly related to fat consumption.

Once again, bacteria in the intestinal tract produce estrogens which fuel cancer growth in such places as the sexual organs. High levels of fat and, especially, cholesterol increase tumor growth as well. Like estrogens, cholesterol acts like a fuel for malignant cells.

Cancer and Protein

A variety of illnesses emerge when protein intake exceeds anywhere from 12 to 17 percent of total calories. Protein is used for cell replacement and repair. When we reach adulthood and stop our physical growth, our need for protein is considerably smaller than our need for energy. Consequently, 75 to 80 percent of our diets should be composed of carbohydrate, with 10 to 15 percent protein, and 10 to 15 percent fat. Unfortunately, because of America's love affair with red meat, dairy foods, and eggs, our protein consumption often exceeds 20 percent, which has been linked with a variety of illnesses, including cancer.

When protein intake exceeds our needs for cell replacement and repair, the body begins to burn protein as fuel. When burned, protein is converted to nitrogen and then to ammonia, which is highly toxic to cells and DNA. Ammonia shortens cell life, alters DNA synthesis, increases our susceptibility to illness, and greatly increases the incidence of tumor growth.

The NRC reported that animal protein seems to enhance tumor growth far more than vegetable protein.

As we showed in the previous chapter, milk products, specifically the sugar found in dairy foods, have been linked to ovarian cancer.

Diet and the Immune System

Saturated fat has been shown to adversely affect the cell membranes of the macrophage and phagocyte cells, the large scavenger cells that patrol the bloodstream looking for foreign objects and pathogens that invade the body. These large white blood cells determine self from not-self by bumping their sensitive cell membrane against foreign objects—everything from dust particles to viruses to cancer cells. Once these cells detect an invader or diseased cell, they gobble it up or mark it with an antigen, which immediately signals the immune system to go into action. The combined immune response is, in most cases, able to wipe out the invading virus or kill the cancer cells, which manifest in all of us from time to time. However, saturated fat coats the membranes of these macrophage and phagocyte cells, causing them to lose their sensitivity and their ability to detect self from not-self. Without their inherent sensitivity, these cells cannot call out the immune system's forces, thus allowing the virus or cancer cells to proliferate and eventually gain a foothold in the organism.

Once inside the system, dietary fat oxidizes, or becomes rancid. As these oxidized fats decay, they cause atoms to lose electrons and form free radicals, highly charged atoms molecules that are extremely reactive and highly destructive to cells and DNA. Once an atom loses one or more electrons, it begins to steal electrons from neighboring atoms. These neighboring atoms, in turn, steal electrons from other atoms, causing chain reactions that destabilize molecules and whole tissues.

As molecules and cells begin to break down, mutations are formed, causing any number of serious illnesses.

Dr. Joe M. McCord, a biochemist at the University of Southern Alabama College of Medicine told *The New York Times* that "the further along we get, the more we are overwhelmed by the number of disease states that involve free radicals." Scientists at the University of Southern Alabama and the University of California at Davis maintain that free radicals are involved in the onset of as many as sixty diseases, including cancer,

Alzheimer's disease, Parkinson's disease, cataracts, arthritis, and immune disorders.

Just as certain foods initiate the free radical process, other foods reverse it. These are called antioxidants, or free radical scavengers, that donate electrons to imbalanced atoms and restore harmony to molecules, cells, and tissues. These antioxidants stop the decaying process that leads to illness. Among the most effective antioxidants are beta-carotene (found in squash, carrots, broccoli, and collard greens), and vitamins C and E. Vitamin C is found in abundance in fruits and vegetables; vitamin E in whole grains and seeds.

In the absence of such nutrients, the immune system must respond to free radicals because they are foreign to healthy human biology. Consequently, the more fat and cholesterol we eat, the more free radical formation takes place. And the more the immune system is called out to deal with the molecular formations and mutant cells that are caused as a result of the free radical formation.

In addition to free radicals, cytotoxins, and fat are the plethora of dietary substances that are foreign to human biology and cause an immune response. These include pesticides, artificial additives, and radioactive nuclides.

Under such conditions, the immune system is continually on red alert, responding to foreign substances, mutant cells, and tissue changes that, if allowed to proliferate, would lead inevitably to disease.

Little wonder that the human race is now faced with a growing list of immune deficiency illnesses, such as Epstein-Barr syndrome and AIDS.

Studies have shown that the strength of the immune system is dependent upon the presence of certain nutrients in the diet, especially zinc, selenium, beta-carotene, manganese, magnesium, copper, calcium, iron, and vitamins C and E. A study published in the *American Journal of Clinical Nutrition* (March 1987) reported that zinc deficiencies caused the atrophy of the thymus gland and reduced the effectiveness of antibodies to fight pathogens. Scientists found that zinc-supplementation strengthened immune response, reduced the number of infections, and increased the number of white blood cells.

Sea vegetables, such as *nori* and *wakame*, provide a nutrient called *sodium alginate*. Studies have shown that sodium alginate binds with radioactive nuclides and chemical pollutants, leaches them from tissues, and brings them to the intestinal tract where they are eliminated from the body. Sea vegetables are one of nature's gifts that cleanse the system.

Clearly, a diet rich in unrefined foods is essential in the maintenance of a healthy immune system. Refined foods, sugar, fat, and cholesterol all act to weaken immune response. Whole foods—low in fat and cholesterol and rich in fiber, vitamins, minerals, and antioxidants—restore and strengthen immune function, and cleanse the body of accumulated waste.

Treating Cancer with Diet

All of this research suggests that diet is essential in the treatment of serious illnesses. And indeed, evidence has been available for decades that shows that diet can play an important role in the treatment of cancer. One of the major themes of this research is that a diet low in fat and cholesterol can dramatically affect tumor growth.

Dr. M.L. Littman showed that when fat and cholesterol are removed from the diet, tumors are reduced to half their original size (*Chemotherapy Reports*, 50: 25–45, 1966).

Other research has shown that cancer cells have higher concentrations of lipids within the cells and exist on cholesterol and fat. Research has shown that lowering cholesterol in the diet retards tumor growth.

Animal studies have shown that tumors in the bowel decrease in size and number when fat and cholesterol are restricted, and fiber is added to the diet. Dr. J.B. Adams showed that breast tumors convert cholesterol to estrogens which fuel cancer growth, and that lowering cholesterol starves tumors by depriving them of estrogens (*Journal of Endocrinology*, 44: 69–77, 1969).

D. G. Jose reported that by lowering protein to below 12 percent of total calories, tumor growth is inhibited (*Medical Tribune*,
5/10/72).

The *New England Journal of Medicine* reported in 1972 a study
by Dr. W. Addelman in which four patients with cancer—three
with prostate cancer and one with ovarian cancer—all experienced
complete remission of their diseases when their cholesterol
levels were dramatically reduced.

Diet has been shown to have a profound effect on immune
response; certain dietary factors can weaken the immune system,
while others strengthen it. In this way, diet can cause illness, or
be used to treat it.

A Macrobiotic Approach to Healing

The macrobiotic approach embraces all these points and goes
several steps further. As we have seen, the macrobiotic diet is
highly effective at lowering blood cholesterol; it provides
moderate levels of protein, and is low in animal protein. Indeed,
as scientists discover more about the relationship between diet
and illness, they unintentionally provide increasing support for
the macrobiotic diet as a means of both prevention and treatment of disease. As a result, it can be used effectively as an
adjunct in cooperation with other medical treatment.

The macrobiotic diet provides an abundance of complex
carbohydrates for long lasting energy; it is rich in the vitamins
and minerals that make for a strong immune system; it provides
a rich supply of antioxidant nutrients; it is extremely low in fat
and cholesterol; it is rich in fiber; and it has been demonstrated
by numerous scientific studies that the macrobiotic diet can be
adhered to.

But as we said, the macrobiotic approach goes beyond the
area of nutrition and into a wider and more holistic understanding.

Specifically, macrobiotics offers two ideas that are essential to
an understanding of human health that are not available in
modern medicine. These include (1) a holistic or unified view of

the human being; and (2) an understanding of how the body eliminates toxins from the system, or a process macrobiotics refers to as discharge.

Toward a Unified View

The philosophy of yin and yang seems obscure and ephemeral at first glance, but with use it is revealed as eminently practical. Indeed, for those involved in healing, yin and yang are as useful to the restoration of health as a carpenter's level is to building a house.

Whether you know it or not, all of us are using yin and yang constantly in our daily lives. A bartender places salty pretzels or chips in front of his patrons because he knows that the salt, which is yang, will cause people to buy more beer or alcohol, which is yin. If one eats more salt and red meat, his or her capacity for alcohol will be greater. After a meal of red meat or chicken, a sweet dessert seems both natural and essential.

We can easily see that stress can be considered a yang condition, in that it causes muscles to contract and our focus to narrow. When we are stressed, our thinking is restricted to our problems; our bodies become tense and either poised for a fight or ready to run from a fight.

Many people who suffer from stress are attracted to sweet foods or alcohol, yin foods that cause one's focus to widen, and the body to relax, temporarily. Sweet foods, such as chocolate, and alcohol can cause a person to temporarily forget his or her immediate issues. Consequently, these foods become highly attractive to people who suffer from a variety of stress-related problems.

Still, there are many healthful ways to deal with imbalance in our lives. When we are suffering from too much stress or yang conditions, we may take a warm bath, or a walk in the woods, or listen to inspiring music, or go dancing—all yin influences. In the end, we are all looking for balance and harmony in our lives, and there are many ways to get it.

The problem with using sugar, alcohol, or drugs as yin influences is that they have powerful side effects. So, too, do excesses of salt, red meat, eggs, or hard cheeses. All of these foods affect our health in extreme ways. These side effects are called illnesses Another way of looking at illness is to see it as forms of imbalance.

Besides having distinct nutritional aspects, each food has its own nature or physical characteristics. While these characteristics can be understood in their material form, as plant or animal cells, they can also be seen abstractly as the movement of cells in a particular direction of growth. The movement that gives rise to a carrot is obviously downward, into the earth; the movement of cells within the collard green plant is upward and fanning outward. Animal foods tend to be more dense, sinewy, and tough than vegetable foods; hence, animal foods are considered more yang than vegetables. Beef is more dense and tough than fish, which tends to be flakey; that is one of the reasons why beef is thought of as more yang than fish.

For the purpose of simplicity, let us consider various vegetables to understand the movement of yin and yang within certain vegetable foods.

In its most abstract form, the growth pattern of a vegetable can be seen as a movement of energy that was ordered by the plant's DNA. This movement or energy gives rise to the pattern of cells that give the plant its own unique design or characteristic form. Thus, each plant has its own distinct characteristics, its own patterning, that arose via the direction of its cells, or—more abstractly—the movement of its energy. Once consumed, each food has a unique effect on the body depending on its characteristic energy.

These energy patterns have been understood by traditional healers in terms of yin and yang.

The human body can be divided into upper and lower, and left and right, outside and inside. Since yin is more expansive and peripheral, we can say that the upper part of the body, from the sternum to the head, is seen as more yin than the lower part, from the sternum to the feet. The skin, or periphery of the body, is more yin than the center of the body, the intestines or, in a man, the prostate, in the woman, the ovaries. In addition, the front part of the body is seen as more yin, or expanded, than the back.

Yin foods and yin influences will cause energy to move upward and outward. Yang foods and yang influences will cause energy to move downward and toward the back of the body. Whole grains are the most balanced food available. Beans and fresh vegetables are also near the center of the yin-yang spectrum, but slightly yin. Fish is slightly yang.

Foods that are more yin, such as yogurt, ice cream, fruit, fruit juice, sugar, alcohol, and (in the extreme) drugs, all affect the upper part of the body, especially the central nervous system, the brain, and the head. For example, sugar will effect the lungs and bronchi; spices, which are yin, will cause headaches; alcohol will effect the liver, nervous system, visual perception, and memory. Drugs are said to be "mind expanding," meaning they have a dramatic effect on the brain and nervous system.

A person with pneumonia, bronchitis, or a brain tumor is suffering from an overly yin condition, brought on by a predominance of yin foods. This person may have eaten steak and hard cheese (more yang foods), too, but he or she indulged excessively in yin foods, as well. In other words, the balance went toward the yin end of the spectrum, much to the detriment of his or her health.

Yang foods, such as salt, red meat, eggs, chicken, fish, and hard cheeses, tend to affect the lower parts of the body, especially the small and large intestines, the kidneys, and sexual organs.

A person with kidney disease, colon or prostate cancer is suffering from an overly yang condition. To be sure, he or she most likely ate sugar and fruits, perhaps, but their tendency was to enjoy more yang foods, such as animal foods, animal fats, baked flour products, salt, and hard cheeses.

In each case, the healing approach is to correct the prevailing imbalance. A person suffering from a yang disease would use a macrobiotic diet that is balanced toward more yin foods. There would be more vegetables, cooked fruit, and foods that include vitamin C (a yin vitamin found in yin foods, such as broccoli and fruits), for example. The cooking should be a little lighter—more steaming, light boiling, less baking and pressure cooking. The person would want to avoid baked products (baking is yang and often includes salt). He or she should also avoid eggs, an excess of salt, red meat, and chicken.

A person suffering from a yin disease would eat a macrobiotic diet that would be slightly balanced toward yang foods, to include more whole grains, root vegetables (carrots, for example, are more yang than, say, collard greens, because they grow downward, into the earth). This is not to say that he or she would avoid collards, broccoli, some cooked fruit, perhaps, and other vegetables. The whole spectrum of the vegetable kingdom would be enjoyed. But there would be an emphasis upon including plenty of grains, roots, and perhaps some fish.

In this way, the philosophy of yin and yang provides us with a compass to help balance our lives. In both yin and yang diseases, a wide variety of foods are employed, but the balance of foods is tilted slightly in one direction or the other, depending on the person's condition. In effect, we are manipulating energy. We are making balance with the prevailing conditions within the person that are giving rise to the illness. By using the macrobiotic diet in this way, we are providing nutritional support for healing, while addressing the underlying, energetic questions of why illnesses manifest where they do. We are using food to make harmony with the energetic imbalances that food produces.

Eliminating Toxins

The typical American diet is characterized by excess—excess fat, cholesterol, calories, unnecessary chemical additives, and sugar. Consequently, accumulation takes place within the body. Atherosclerosis builds within the arteries; fat builds in the tissues; and dietary and environmental chemical pollutants accumulate in fat cells. Because the diet is so rich, this accumulation continues through much of our lives.

When we adopt a macrobiotic diet, we begin to eliminate this

accumulated buildup. As we saw in the previous chapter, cholesterol plaque can be eliminated, or—as traditional healers would
say—"discharged," from the body. So, too, can excess fat and
accumulated toxins, such as radioactive nuclides and chemical
pollutants. To do this, the diet must nourish the body efficiently
without adding excess. When the diet itself is free of waste, the
liver and kidneys can begin cleansing the blood of stored toxins.
Atherosclerosis in the arteries and tissues can be discharged, as
well as foreign chemicals. A cleansing process takes place.

Part of this cleansing process includes the common cold. While
medical professionals view the cold as a disease and a hindrance
to be snuffed out, the macrobiotic view is that the cold is a
natural process that the body employs to eliminate accumulated
waste in the blood, lymph, sinuses, and tissues. The common cold
is actually the body's way of house cleaning. To eliminate the
common cold—which is to say, to depress the symptoms of the
cold—is to eliminate an important method of cleansing the
system.

Thus, the macrobiotic view of healing is three-fold: to nourish
the body optimally and enhance immune function; to restore
balance or harmony to the mind, body, and spirit; and to
eliminate—as much as possible—those constituents that accumulate and inevitably lead to illness; this is done by eliminating
such toxins from the diet, which leads in turn to the elimination
of accumulated toxins from the body. By performing all three
tasks, the macrobiotic approach allows the underlying strength
of the body—the body's own recuperative powers—to be directed
toward the illness, rather than dealing additionally with the daily
onslaught of poisons that are typically consumed in the standard
American diet.

Adult-onset Diabetes

So far, we have talked about cardiovascular disease, including
coronary heart disease and high blood pressure, and various
types of cancer. We have shown how diet causes these illnesses
and how it can be used to reverse them. We have also shared

with you how diet influences our immune system for good or ill, and how we can eat to make our immune system stronger. Now, let us turn our attention to diabetes, the third leading cause of death in the United States, and a leading killer disease in the industrialized world.

Diabetes attacks some 12 million Americans today, 11 million of whom are considered adult-onset diabetics. About a million diabetics are considered type I, or juvenile diabetics, meaning that their pancreas no longer secretes adequate quantities of insulin to support life. Insulin is a hormone that is utilized by the body to metabolize sugar, which the body uses for fuel. Without insulin, the body's cells do not get fuel, and without fuel, cells die. Juvenile diabetics usually experience rapid weight loss and require insulin in order to survive.

Type II diabetes, also known as adult-onset, usually occurs later in life.

Both types of diabetes are associated with a number of other serious illnesses, including cardiovascular disease, blindness, gangrene, progressive loss of hearing, impotence, and palsy. There have been numerous misconceptions about diabetes, especially adult-onset diabetes, or type II, through most of this century.

Scientists believed for many years that adult-onset diabetics were unable to produce sufficient quantities of insulin to sustain health. Consequently, doctors gave them insulin injections or oral medication. Both of these are still administered.

Along with the drugs, doctors told diabetics to avoid eating carbohydrates, even complex carbohydrates from whole grains, vegetables, and fruits, which were thought to be harmful to diabetics because carbohydrates are sugars, which the diabetic has trouble metabolizing. Consequently, doctors prescribed a high protein, high fat diet, rich in red meats, dairy products, and eggs. Doctors thought a high fat diet was not particularly a problem for diabetics. Carbohydrates was the problem, they believed.

But in 1970, scientists learned that type II diabetics were in fact producing insulin, and sometimes they were producing more insulin than non-diabetics. The problem was that the insulin was not able to make sufficient quantities of glucose, or blood sugar, available to cells. Something was going wrong in the process of utilizing insulin to make sugar available to cells.

Meanwhile, studies had existed for decades showing that carbohydrates were not the cause of diabetes; fat was the cause.

In 1935, Dr. H.P. Himsworth discovered that you could make a healthy adult diabetic simply by putting him or her on a high fat diet. After one week of a high fat diet, the person would test diabetic. Himsworth also found that he could reverse the process and restore health by placing the same person on a low fat diet.

One of the first people to recognize this connection between fat and diabetes was Nathan Pritikin, the self-taught nutritionist. He theorized that dietary fat coats the cells and prevents insulin from attaching to specific places on the cell, called *insulin receptor sites*. It is here, at the insulin receptor sites, that insulin allows glucose to enter the cell. When these insulin receptor sites are closed off by fat, glucose cannot penetrate the cell, thus starving the cell for fuel.

Pritikin demonstrated that adult-onset diabetics could be cured with the use of a low fat, low cholesterol diet made up of whole grains and vegetables.

Recent research done during the 1970s and 1980s by Dr. James Anderson at the University of Kentucky Medical School proved Pritikin's hypothesis. Anderson demonstrated that a high fat diet does indeed give rise to a diabetic state, and that a low fat, high fiber diet can reverse adult-onset diabetes and restore blood sugar levels to normal.

Following Anderson's research and other studies that confirmed the findings, the American Diabetics Association began recommending that diabetics eat a low fat, low cholesterol diet that is rich in whole grains, vegetables, and fiber. While insulin and oral medication are still prescribed, diabetics—especially adult-onset diabetics—are encouraged to eat a diet low in fat and rich in fiber. This diet has been shown to reverse type II, adult-onset diabetes.

It has also been shown to protect diabetics against many of the related illnesses, such as blindness, gangrene, and athero-sclerosis.

Juvenile diabetics do not produce sufficient insulin to metabolize sugar and thus need insulin injections. But they, too, should avoid a high fat diet in order to protect themselves against the related illnesses that so commonly afflict diabetics.

Gout and Other Forms of Arthritis

Gout is a painful joint pain that has been shown to afflict people who consume diets rich in animal proteins. Gout was especially prevalent among the aristocracy of the seventeenth century England, when the rich ate meat in various forms at least three times per day. Since Westerners are consuming animal products in unrivaled quantities, gout and other forms of arthritis have surfaced once again.

The problem with gout is uric acid, a by-product of protein metabolism. High protein diets cause uric acid levels in the blood to increase. Uric acid can crystalize in the joints where it is treated by the immune system as a foreign object. The white blood cell attempts to consume the uric acid crystal in its acid-rich stomach, which is called a *lysosome*. But the crystal cannot be digested by the white blood cell and, instead, sometimes punctures a hole in the cell, causing the acid to spill out onto the joints and sensitive joint tissues. This gives rise to the associated pain.

By eliminating high protein foods, especially animal foods, gout can be eliminated.

Other forms of arthritis are often relieved in the same way. Animal proteins, of course, come with fat, which reduces circulation and oxygen levels in joints. Blood and oxygen are essential for tissues to function properly. As fat and cholesterol increase in the blood, the rouleaux formation takes place (explained in Chapters 2 and 3), causing sludging of red blood cells, edema, and swelling of joints. A macrobiotic diet increases circulation, reduces uric acid levels and its crystals, and brings optimal levels of oxygen to suffocating joint tissues. The macrobiotic approach also encourages arthritis-sufferers to avoid acidic foods, especially tomatoes and eggplant. Acid seems to play a role creating greater number of crystals and reducing oxygen. Coupling highly acidic foods with those that are high in fat, cholesterol, and protein, arthritis symptoms quickly escalate. However, by avoiding these foods, blood circulation and oxygen in the joints increase significantly and cause the elimination of arthritis symptoms.

Many Disease States One Disease

What we have seen is that many illnesses emerge from a single cause: our daily eating patterns. Foods that we have come to take for granted are poisoning us. But we can reverse their poisonous effects by changing our way of eating. Whole grains, fresh vegetables, beans, sea vegetables, fruits, and fish all enhance the underlying strength of the human body. Our bodies have been designed by nature to deal effectively with the antagonisms of our environment, including disease. We were made to be well. By supporting the body's natural defenses, we can recover our health. Macrobiotics does not heal; the body heals; macrobiotics merely facilitates the body's healing mechanisms.

Chapter 6
Getting Old and Dying, Western Style

In central Mexico, a tribe of Indians called the Tarahumara play a game that makes the celebrated 26-mile marathon run look like a walk in the park. The Tarahumara's game is to run and kick a ball for 100 miles. That is right—100 miles! And the only time a play stops running is to urinate. The Tarahumara women play the same game, but they only run for 60 miles. Dr. William Connor, one of the world's preeminent cardiovascular researchers, studied the Tarahumara Indians and discovered that it is not uncommon for the men to be able to run 200 miles.

The Tarahumara eat a very simple diet composed almost entirely of whole grains, vegetables, and fruits. They rarely eat meat or dairy products. These Indians have no sign of heart disease or other degenerative illnesses. Moreover, they have tremendous stamina and vitality well into old age.

The human body is capable of many remarkable feats. In the modern industrialized world, our definition of our own limits is shaped, in part, by what we have come to take for granted: that aging means becoming increasingly dependent upon drugs, surgery, high-tech medicine, relatives and institutions. But when we examine more traditional cultures, cultures that subsist on more simple eating, we see is a very different picture: people do not get high blood pressure, osteoporosis, strokes or heart attacks as a consequence of aging. In fact, in traditional cultures, blood pressures remain stable and even decline somewhat with age; osteoporosis is rare, as is angina pectoris; in short, they do not suffer from the pandemic rates of heart attack, stroke, or cancer. Instead, there is a high degree of vitality and clarity well into old age. There is not the dependence upon drugs, surgery, and technology in the senior years.

In the modern industrialized world, people in their 50s, 60s, and 70s have become—to one degree or another—functionally dependent. They must rely on drugs, various surgical procedures and technological apparatuses to sustain their biological functions, and sometimes even to stay alive. The old age we see in the West is a social burden, a time when many suffer from the steady loss of sight, hearing, physical strength, and mental clarity.

We have come to take this state of affairs for granted, but it need not be so.

Spending a Lifetime Getting Sick

The process of contracting heart disease, cancer, high blood pressure, adult-onset diabetes, arthritis, and obesity, and the loss of the senses is a lifelong endeavor. It creeps up on us and gains greater control of our lives with each passing day. It moves so insidiously that we stop noticing it *because the process is our way of life*. It is so familiar that it seems to be the only way to live. But it is a *degeneration* process. The effects of the toxins in our diets—especially fat and cholesterol—build over time so that more and more of our energy goes toward sustaining life, rather than toward the fulfillment of our dreams. Slowly, ever so slowly, we become less effective, less alert, physically and mentally weaker, until finally we are struck down by a heart attack, or cancer, or some other crippling illness.

Actually, the sickness itself is the result of our lifelong habits, many of which could have been changed earlier in life. Those habits finally manifest as an illness. But these diseases are the fruits of our learned behavior.

It seems to many as if the disease came suddenly. People say: "He wasn't sick a day in his life. What happened?" The answer is that *he was sick everyday of his life*, but he was so strong that his body was able to keep the illness at bay. Scientists at the American Heart Association tell us that heart disease begins before a child reaches the age of ten. He or she may not have a heart attack until the age of fifty, but the cause of the illness began before puberty.

You may argue that we, in the West, have excellent longevity, but think about that for a second: What is the quality of life for most old people today? The vast majority of senior citizens today are dependent upon medication or technology to support their vital functions. They take medication to maintain heart rate, control hypertension, angina or arthritis pain, slow the loss of bone, treat cataracts or glaucoma, or deal with adult-onset diabetes. A sizable portion of the senior population is over-weight and many are obese. Such illnesses as angina pectoris (the characteristic pain in the chest related to heart disease), arthritis, and hearing loss are so common that they are taken for granted. Nursing homes are overcrowded. Many seniors are left to spend the rest of their remaining days almost comatose. Meanwhile, degenerative brain diseases, such as Alzheimer's and Parkinson's diseases, are ravaging the senior population. Cancer rates continue to climb, despite the much ballyhooed "War on Cancer," and heart disease remains the leading killer in the Western world. Among the very modern issues facing us today is the "right to die." Many people today do not want to be kept alive by technological and pharmaceutical means. None of these indicators represent health and vitality in old age. On the contrary, they represent a "false longevity," another cause in which statistics lie. You may live to be sixty-five or seventy, but do you want that kind of life? For most of us, the unequivocal answer is "No."

Yet, when we examine pre-modern or the so-called primitive populations, you find a high incidence of vitality, clarity, and fully functioning senior citizens. Few are dependent in any way on drugs or surgery or high-tech equipment. These people are free of osteoporosis and hip fractures. You may argue that a sizable portion of the pre-modern senior citizens are dead before they reach sixty-five, but that is not true. The average forty year old man living in Bolivia has a greater chance of living to seventy-three than the average forty year old American man. People in pre-modern cultures do not get old and die like those of us in the West do. You do not find the incidence of senility, hearing loss, diabetes, arthritis, coronary disease, or cancer among the senior populations in pre-modern cultures. Let us look at some of the most common illnesses prevalent among senior citizens today, and examine their link to the high fat, high cholesterol diet.

Sure you can listen, but can you hear?

In the West, we experience a steady loss of hearing that cannot be found among traditional peoples of any age.

Researchers compared the hearing capabilities of people living in Wisconsin, the dairy capital of the United States, with the African tribe's people, called the Mabaans. The scientists found that the hearing loss among young Wisconsin people between the ages of thirty to thirty-five was worse than anything that could be found among the Mabaans, at any age. In other words, the degree of hearing loss that was common among young Wisconsinites could not be found among even the oldest African tribesmen.

Researchers randomly selected a population of young people from Finland, ages ten to nineteen, and discovered that they had lost the capacity to hear sounds at 16,000 to 18,000 cycles per second, a range of sound commonly heard in all pre-modern cultures. When the researchers examined the same age groups in Yugoslavia, no such hearing loss was discovered.

Research has shown that atherosclerosis clogs the tiny arteries that nourish the hearing mechanism of the inner ear, thus making the ear less sensitive to sound as the atherosclerosis worsens. Other research has shown that by lowering the fat and cholesterol content of the diet, the atherosclerosis can be reversed and lost hearing can be recovered.

Seeing is believing.

Much of the impaired sight in the West is caused by poor blood circulation to the eye. A common occurrence among Americans forty years and older is the appearance of a semicircular plaque that develops around the iris of the eye called *arcus senilis*, or arc of age. This plaque is caused by cholesterol that collects within the eye and forms a hard growth around the iris. According to the *American Medical Association's Encyclopedia of Medicine*, arcus senilis "occurs almost invariably during old age." Arcus senilis also appears in children sometimes, and, according to the AMA, "this condition may be associated with the metabolic disorder *hyperlipidemia*," or high levels of lipids or cholesterol and fat in the blood.

Atherosclerosis causes cholesterol plaques to form throughout the body, including the eye. Pieces of these plaques often break off and float in the bloodstream. These fragments of plaque can become lodged in the eye; under examination, ophthalmologists can see them floating in the lens and cornea of the eye. These fragments of plaque, which exist as crystals, can block blood flow to the eye and impair sight and ultimately cause blindness.

Vision can be impaired in yet another way: by changing interocular pressure within the eye, which causes a disease called *glaucoma*. The eye is continually being nourished by fluids that contain nutrients and oxygen that pass from the blood into the lens of the eye by osmosis. Waste in the form of carbon dioxide, cell debris, and cholesterol drain from the lens via a canal-like passageway. This inflow and outflow of fluids maintains the pressure within the eye, and thus is kept in balance. Blood containing high levels of fat and cholesterol can cause changes in eye pressure by backing up the outflow of waste and fluids or by increasing the pressure of incoming fluids.

Once pressure is changed within the eye, the range of vision narrows. This narrowing of vision is characteristic of glaucoma.

Since all cells depend upon the availability of blood and oxygen, lack of blood flow to other parts of the eye, such as the retina or optic nerve, can cause visual changes as well. Consequently, circulation to the eye is essential for proper sight.

Nathan Pritikin, who, in addition to being an expert nutritionist, also possessed a deep understanding of the eye, believed that at least half of all impaired vision was caused by the typical high fat diet of Western industrialized nations.

Senility: The Source of Old Age

Much of the senility experienced in old age is due to insufficient blood supply to the brain. That loss of blood supply is caused by atherosclerosis. By reducing blood flow to the brain, brain cells become impaired and many die, thus causing a severe diminution of mental faculties later in life. Once again, the incidence of senility among many pre-modern populations is low in comparision to that of the West.

Osteoporosis: Simply Getting More Calcium Is Not the Answer

Approximately 20 million American women suffer from osteoporosis, or porous bones. A much smaller but still significant number of men also suffer from the illness. Osteoporosis causes bone fractures, particularly in the spine, wrist, leg, and hip. Apart from being traumatic and life altering, these fractures can, in older adults, lead to death. Osteoporosis is a fast growing illness throughout the modern, industrialized world. Ironically, it is also a recent illness, having arisen in such numbers only within the last three decades.

There are four main risk factors in the onset of osteoporosis.

1. Genes. Blacks tend to suffer fewer cases of osteoporosis than whites, men fewer than women.
2. Diet.
3. Lack of exercise and movement in general.
4. Being a woman. Women experience radical loss of bone, especially after thirty years of age. Osteoporosis increases rapidly after menopause, when women lose the ability to produce estrogen, which is an essential hormone in the production of bone material.

Ironically, studies have shown that traditional peoples do not suffer osteoporosis at anywhere near the rates that are common in modern, industrialized nations. Bantu women of New Guinea, for example, bear and nurse more than six children on the average and show no loss of bone later in life. They eat a diet that is primarily whole grains, vegetables, fruits, and small amounts of animal foods. Their average daily intake of calcium is approximately 400 to 500 milligrams, while the U.S. recommended daily allowance is 1,000 milligrams.

As we have already seen in the previous chapter, the Chinese people get only half the calcium Americans do, but do not suffer from the osteoporosis rates that we do in the United States.

According to Dr. Robert Lang, a former assistant professor at the Yale Medical School and a leading expert on osteoporosis, studies have shown that several factors within the typical Western diet contribute to bone loss. Among these are the following:

1. The consumption of high quantities of animal proteins, from red meat, chicken, dairy products, and eggs. Animal proteins bind with calcium and cause greater quantities of calcium to be excreted through the kidneys.
2. Excess consumption of foods rich in phosphates, such as dairy products. Phosphates are composed of phosphorus, oxygen, and salts that are essential to calcium absorption but in high quantities tend to interfere with calcium uptake.
3. Excess consumption of insoluble fiber. Insoluble fiber, found especially in wheat, contains phytates, which can initially interfere with calcium absorption in some people. However, studies have shown that the human body adapts to insoluble fiber and the presence of phytates, and overcomes an initial tendency of phytates to disrupt calcium absorption. Dr. Lang encourages people to eat a diet composed chiefly of whole grains and vegetables and low in animal products. However, he tries to dissuade people from eating bran as a supplement to the diet because of the presence of phytates.
4. Excess consumption of salt. Excess salt intake tends to bind with calcium and leach the mineral from the body, through the kidneys.

5. Excess consumption of caffeine. Caffeine has been shown to interfere with calcium absorption.

6. Excess consumption of sugar. Sugar interferes with trace mineral absorption, thereby limiting the body's ability to take in calcium.

7. Excess consumption of alcohol. Alcohol shrinks sexual organs and creates hormonal imbalances that prevent the utilization of calcium by the bones.

8. Excess consumption of vitamin D. Vitamin D is essential in the absorption of calcium for bones and teeth. However, excess intake of vitamin D increases calcium utilization, which ultimately leads to diminished quantities of calcium in tissues and bone. According to Dr. Lang, fifteen to twenty minutes of sunlight each day is sufficient to provide optimal quantities of vitamin D.

9. Diets too low or too high in calcium. Proper calcium balance in the diet is essential to the body's ability to absorb calcium. Diets deficient in calcium will lead to bone loss. Interestingly, diets containing excess quantities of calcium will also impair the body's ability to utilize calcium, studies have shown.

In order to maintain the health of bones, exercise is essential. Dr. Lang says that daily walking or twenty minutes a day of simple stretching exercises are sufficient to maintain healthy bones.

Other factors that contribute to bone loss include excess stress, which causes hormonal imbalances that prevent optimal utilization of calcium.

For people who want to prevent osteoporosis or restore lost bone matter, Dr. Lang recommends a diet of whole grains, fresh leafy green vegetables, beans, small quantities of sea vegetables, and small amounts of animal foods, especially fish and the bones of fish, which are rich in calcium.

Leafy green vegetables are loaded with calcium and other trace minerals. So, too, are sea vegetables. Grains contain minerals, including calcium. And the bones of fish are one of the richest sources of calcium available.

We have shown that the major diseases facing us today are related in one way or another to a diet rich in fat and cholesterol, sugar, refined grains, and artificial ingredients. The biggest poisons of all are fat and cholesterol. These two affect us in ways that are more deleterious than any other food substances available. But the other toxins in the diet can also be extremely dangerous and damaging to health.

The human body is capable of many marvelous things, especially when it is fed properly and exercised regularly. Let us turn our attention now to exercise and then have a look at the diet that can change your life—for the better.

Chapter 7

Exercise: The Blessing
of That Little Walk Every Day

**I hate exercise and I hate to think about it because it makes me
feel so guilty. What can I do to get out of this trap?**

The first thing you need to know is that a little bit of exercise
goes a long, long way. You do not have to become a well-trained
athlete to benefit from exercise. In fact, the research shows just
the opposite: the greatest protection against disease comes to
those who go from being sedentary to taking as a brisk half-hour
walk every day.

In November 1989, the *Journal of the American Medical
Association* reported a study conducted by the Institute for
Aerobic Research in Dallas in which 13,344 men and women
were followed for eight years to determine what effect, if any,
fitness had on mortality rates. The participants were divided into
five groups, from least fit to most fit. Fitness was measured
directly by having each participant walk on a treadmill. The
incline and speed of the treadmill were increased periodically to
increase fitness. People were categorized into levels of fitness
according to how well they performed on the treadmill test. (This
was the first study that measured fitness directly, rather than
basing its evaluation on questionnaires.)

After eight years of following the participants, the scientists
discovered that death rates were dramatically higher among the
least fit.

What was surprising was that the greatest difference in mortality existed between the least fit people—those in the first level
of fitness—compared to those who were in the next level up in
fitness, or the second level of fitness. Comparing these two
groups, the death rate was three times higher among the least fit

than those in the second level of fitness. In other words, the scientists discovered that small differences in fitness created enormous differences in health and longevity.

This was a remarkable discovery, since the scientists had expected to find that the high intensity athletes—men and women who ran 30 to 40 miles per week—would show the most dramatic differences in mortality rate. But this was not the case.

By counting the number of people who died in each of the five categories of fitness, the scientists were able to extrapolate the number of people who would die annually in each fitness group, if each group had 10,000 people in it.

The results showed that 64 deaths per 10,000 people occur each year in the least fit, while only 25.5 deaths per 10,000 people occur in the second level of fitness. The third level showed 27.1 deaths per 10,000 people; the fourth level of fitness showed 21.7 deaths per 10,000 people, and the fifth level of fitness—the most well-trained athletes in the group—showed 18.6 deaths per 10,000 people.

"Even modest amounts of exercise can substantially reduce a person's chances of dying" of heart disease, cancer, and other illnesses, reported *The New York Times* (November 3, 1989).

"This is a hopeful message, an important message for the American people to understand," Dr. Carl Caspersen of the Federal Centers for Disease Control told *The New York Times*. "You don't have to be a marathoner. In fact, you get much more benefit out of being just a bit more active. For example, going from being sedentary to walking briskly for a half hour several days a week can drop your risk dramatically."

Another of the study's remarkable findings was that this moderate amount of exercise substantially reduced the risk of all causes of death, particularly heart disease and cancer, the two leading killer diseases. Scientists speculated that the protection exercise provides against heart disease stemmed from its tendency to increase circulation to the heart. However, they were not sure why moderate exercise protects against cancer.

It has been known for decades that diminution of oxygen to tissues increases the likelihood of cancer. Exercise increases oxygen to tissues throughout the body, and in this way may decrease the chances of malignancy.

The study demonstrated that the most significant benefits from exercise came from the smallest investment of time and energy— a half-hour to an hour walk several times per week was enough to dramatically decrease mortality rates, the study showed. Just getting out of the sedentary lifestyle improves one's health and longevity.

Many of the physiological benefits from aerobic exercise have been recognized for some time. Aerobic exercises, such as walking, running, bicycling, swimming, jumping jacks, knee bends and toe touching, all increase the intake of oxygen (hence the name aerobic). They increase the speed of the heartbeat, improve circulation to tissues throughout the body, stretch muscles, and speed elimination of carbon dioxide, uric acid, and other forms of waste stored in the tissues.

By causing the heart to beat faster, exercise makes the heart work more efficiently. Its expansion and contraction occurs in a more coordinated fashion. In this way, the heart is able to take in more blood during its expansive phase, or diastole, and pump greater quantities of blood in a single contraction during its systole phase.

By making the heart work more efficiently, you are actually causing the heart to rest more frequently. The average man's heart beats at a rate of seventy-two beats per minute, the average woman's at seventy-six beats per minute. As heartbeat slows down, the time between beats is extended. The difference between sixty beats per minute and ninety is that the heart rests twice as long between beats.

Exercise lowers blood pressure, as well. It does this in part by opening vessels and by creating new circulation. As one increases exercise, muscle tissues throughout the body must work harder and consequently demand more oxygen. In order to provide more oxygen, the body grows new blood vessels so that more blood and oxygen can be transported to cells. Exercises also reduce the stickiness between blood platelets, which causes sludging of the blood and diminishes blood flow. (Exercise will not lower your cholesterol level or reverse atherosclerosis, however; only your low fat, low cholesterol diet will do that.)

Any exercise that involves the legs—such as walking or bicycling—improves circulation because the leg muscles act as auxilary pumps. Their expansion and contraction causes blood to be pumped through the vessels and back to the heart. This substantially reduces the burden on the heart.

Exercise also improves circulation to the brain and helps to dissolve blood clots throughout the body that might otherwise cause a heart attack or stroke.

Exercise increases the body's demand for fuel and thus burns stored calories. In this way, it reduces weight by using carbohydrates from the diet and burning body fat.

Exercise also strengthens bones in two ways: the first is that it increases bone growth and mass; the second way is by strengthening muscles, thereby decreasing the stress on the bone. Exercise has been shown to decrease the number of bone fractures.

Muscles and bones that are not exercised begin to atrophy. One of the major causes of bone loss (osteoporosis) and fractures is a sedentary lifestyle, or the lack of exercise.

The benefits of exercise to the mind are also well documented. The natural "high" runners talk about is the secretion of beta endorphines in the brain. These morphine-like chemicals cause a deep sense of well-being and are a natural antidote to depression and anxiety.

The Greatest Exercise of All

> I have met but one or two persons in the course of my life who understood the art of walking, that is, of taking walks—who had a genius, so to speak, for *sauntering*.
> —Henry David Thoreau
> (from his essay, *Walking*)

Humans were built to walk. It is the best exercise there is and it is free for the taking. It should not even be called exercise—for *exercise* is a modern word that separates us from the joy of this, a human's most natural means of locomotion. For those who are not handicapped, walking is a blessing.

Still, walking is a wonderful exercise, and a half-hour's worth of walking conditions the entire body. With arms swinging and legs stepping freely according to your own pace, you are exercising your muscles, heart, respiratory and circulatory systems, without even thinking of the fact that you are exercising. Walking seems to lighten the load, it provides perspective while it works off the tension generated by stressful thoughts.

Walking in nature is the ideal because the trees and plants pump out so much oxygen and provide such a healing and relaxing atmosphere. The calm of nature is infectious. It sooths the body and mind; walking in nature provides a kind of massage for the soul.

But if you cannot walk in a local park or wood, you can still lose yourself on the city streets or by trekking around your own block.

Walk at a brisk pace, but do not go beyond your capacity. Rest whenever you need to, and follow by taking up a pace that is comfortable. Walking briskly is not jogging or running. Brisk walks are those that maintain a pace just beyond a comfortable stroll. As your conditioning improves, you can increase your speed. But start out slowly and work up to a faster pace as you gain conditioning and confidence. (People who have not exercised are advised to see their physician before taking up any exercise program.)

For those of you who are ready to improve their fitness a little more rapidly, all you need to do is walk briskly for thirty minutes or take three ten-minute bursts four times per week. If you can maintain a brisk pace longer, all the better. But do not strain yourself, particularly if you have not exercised in a while.

In-between each brisk ten-minute burst, you can rest or stroll. The routine can be a brisk walk for ten minutes; rest or stroll for a while, and then do two more intervals of ten minutes each, with whatever rest is needed in-between. Once you have done these stretches, you have done all that you need to do for that day's exercise. You have begun to condition your body. You will find that your conditioning will improve steadily and you will be surprised at how different your body feels in a couple of weeks of regular walking.

For those who are interested in heart rates and conditioning, exercise experts tell us that in order to condition the heart, you must get your pulse rate up to 120 beats per minute for at least two minutes. The heart has a maximum capacity of 220 beats per minute. Once the heart rate has reached that peak, it will not go any faster, no matter how much more strenuously you exercise.

However, people who are not in good health or are not well-conditioned should avoid stressing their heart unduly, especially at the beginning of a new program. Rest whenever you feel you need to. The beauty of walking is that very few people go beyond their capacity and consequently walking rarely causes any real discomfort or serious side effects. For example, heart attacks while walking are rare, but much more frequent while running.

Here are some ideas for starting an exercise program, and keeping it going.

Make your intention clear: All you are looking for is fun.
Remember that the best exercise is fun. Unless your intention is to become a highly conditioned, competitive athlete, your true goal is to enjoy your life. Being fit is a way to better enjoy your body and your life in general. Becoming fit should not be painful or unpleasant. We all are little children at heart and the last thing we want to do with our leisure hours is torture our bodies for whatever delusion that may be afflicting us of late. Such things rarely if ever last, as most of us have learned at one time or another. Forget about looking like Charles Atlas or Barbie. Instead, eat well and have fun; your appearance will improve dramatically, and without effort, and the glow of your smile will attract friends and lovers from near and far.

Pick a safe place and time to walk and do it at least four times per week. It is free, it does not require a partner, and the only equipment you need are some comfortable shoes and loose clothing.

Walk with a friend. Walking is cheap therapy. Walk with your spouse, friend, or lover and get to know each other better. Also, someone from your neighborhood might love to get into a routine for walking at a particular hour of the day. Think about it.

Take up dancing. Aerobic dancing was the craze during the 1980s and is still available to most everyone. Begin slowly and gradually increase the level of intensity as your conditioning improves. Do not tax yourself excessively, especially in the beginning.

Join a club. Lots of towns have organized nature walks and hiking clubs. Walking with others is a chance to make new friends and have fun while you are exercising. Consult your local recreation department for organizations that provide regular walking clubs or hiking programs.

Join the YMCA or YWMC. The YMCA or YWCA provides everything from swimming to basketball to volleyball to hiking. Call the Y or drop by and talk to the nice people there about the programs being offered and see what works for you.

Private instructors offer on-going classes in yoga, stretching, and other forms of exercise. These clubs and classes are usually very inexpensive and are great ways to socialize while you exercise. Consult the newspaper or your town's recreation department for the whereabouts and times for such classes.

If you can afford it and you are sufficiently fit, join a fitness, racketball, tennis, or golf club or take lessons in one or another of these sports.

Ride a bike. One of the greatest and most enjoyable exercises you will ever experience on this earth. Bicycling is highly aerobic.

It can also be a very demanding conditioning program. People are advised to start out slowly and gradually work up to greater distances or hillier terrains.

Before you buy a bicycle, talk to someone who knows bikes. Tell him or her where you will be riding most of the time—in parks, on paved roads, or off-the road. The bike-shop person will fit you correctly for a bike, depending on your height and weight. Once you have got a bicycle, start out on a flat terrain and avoid hills or irregular surfaces until you have grown stronger and more accustomed to riding.

Bicycling is addictive; once you get into the habit of bike riding, you will be out every morning or evening, weather permitting, of course.

If not a two-wheeler, than a stationary bike. Stationary bikes are among the most popular forms of exercise available today. One of the benefits of a stationary bike is that you do not have to look where you are going. People who use stationary bikes often listen to music, self-help tapes, and meditate themselves into tranquility.

Avoid competitive games, especially if you are out of shape. If you are new to exercise, it is wise to avoid competitive games because people often forget themselves in the heat of battle. The consequence for many is a fatal heart attack.

If you take up tennis or some other strenuous game, see a physician first and engage in some other less strenuous exercise program, such as brisk walking, to improve your conditioning before you engage in any competitive sport.

Brand new tennis players should spend a few weeks rallying and allowing your body to get used to the demands of exercise. Rallying alone will condition your heart and body, and will be lots of fun. Also, begin each session with a set of warm-up exercises, especially stretching.

Senior citizens and people out of condition can enjoy a variety of exercises grounded in Oriental philosophy, such as Dō-In, a self-massage technique, or Tai Chi, a martial art that is performed as a beautiful and graceful dance. Classes are provided for these and other meditative exercises in many cities and towns. Consult your Yellow Pages, call your recreation department, or an adult education department at a local college.

There are lots of ways to be physically fit, and most of them can be fun. In fact, the only way to be fit is to maintain your program consistently, and the only way to maintain consistency is to enjoy yourself.

Chapter 8

The Macrobiotic Diet:
The Whole and Its Parts

Macrobiotics is a way of establishing health and harmony in daily life. The most basic part of the macrobiotic approach is its dietary program, which includes whole grains, beans, land and sea vegetables as its principal foods. The diet also contains a variety of soups, pickles, condiments, seasonings, beverages, fruits, and fish. The proportion of each food one consumes is determined by one's own health and goals in life.

For most people living in a temperate climate, the diet is composed of approximately 50 percent whole grains, 25 to 30 percent vegetables, 10 percent beans and sea vegetables, and the remainder composed of soups, condiments, fish, fruit, desserts, and snacks. The specific foods are outlined below.

Whole Grains

Whole grains are exactly that: the whole cereal grain before it has been stripped of its fiber, protein, and mineral content. Refined grains, found in white bread and white flour products, have been processed so that the fiber and germ are removed. The germ contains protein, vitamins, and minerals.

Harvard University agronomist professor Paul C. Manglesdorf says this about whole grains: "A whole grain cereal, if its food values are not destroyed by the overrefining of modern processing methods, comes closer than any other plant product to providing an adequate diet. No civilization worthy of its name has never been founded on any agricultural basis other than [whole grain] cereals."

We are not recommending that one eat only whole cereal

grains. On the contrary, a varied diet is essential to good health and the key to the full enjoyment of our food.

But the center of our diet should be whole cereal grains. Grain is the staple of life, the basis upon which human health has been founded.

Brown rice

Brown rice comes in three varieties: short, medium, and long grain. Short grain is consumed most frequently, but medium and long grain may be preferred during hot summer months.

Brown rice is rich in complex carbohydrates, potassium, phosphorus, B vitamins, and niacin. It contains protein, iron, and other minerals. Like all whole grains, brown rice is low in fat.

Brown rice is prepared by pressure cooking and boiling. It is cooked with a pinch of sea salt or a stalk of *kombu*. It can be combined with other grains, such as millet, barley, or with beans, such as *azuki* beans.

Sweet brown rice

The more glutenous form of brown rice. Rich in protein and all the nutrients common to brown rice, sweet rice can be cooked with beans, such as azuki, to make a rich, and hearty bean-and-grain dish.

Barley

Barley—both as whole grain and its slightly refined form, "pearled" barley—contains phosphorus, magnesium, potassium and B vitamins. Barley is wonderful in soups, stews, cooked with a variety of other hearty vegetables and beans, such as carrots, onions, chick-peas, navy, and pinto beans. It is delicious when cooked in a miso or tamari broth.

Mochi

Mochi is pounded sweet rice, very hearty and strengthening. Available in natural stores, prepackaged and ready to cook.

Millet
Can be boiled or pressure cooked by itself, or cooked with a variety of vegetables, especially cauliflower, carrots, and other grains, such as barley or rice.

Oats
Oats come as whole, steel-cut, or rolled. Boiled as a breakfast cereal, oats can be combined with a variety of fruits or eaten plain.

Whole wheat
Whole wheat berries; whole wheat bread; chapatis, whole wheat noodles, including *udon*, bulgur, *fu* (baked puffed wheat gluten), *seitan* (kneeded wheat gluten, meaty and hearty).

Noodles
There are a wide variety of nutritious whole grain or partially refined noodles, including udon, a rich and delicious spaghetti-like noodle; whole wheat pastas; *soba*, or buckwheat noodles; various combined-flours, such as whole wheat and buckwheat, and *jinenjo* noodles, which combines the jinenjo potato with whole wheat flour.

Buckwheat
Buckwheat can be used as groats, noodles, and flour products, such as pancakes. Buckwheat is a hearty grass used as a grain, especially in winter because it has a warming effect on the body. It can be cooked with sauerkraut and a variety of vegetables, including carrots and onions.

Cooking Grains

Grains can be pressure-cooked, boiled, steamed, fried, and baked. Use small amounts (small pinch) of sea salt when cooking grains to help break the fiber coating and make them easier to digest.

Vegetables

A wide variety of vegetables are a necessity in a healthful diet. The vegetable kingdom provides such a wealth of nutrients (see nutrients section below) that to avoid them is to guarantee the undermining of your health. They are rich in vitamins, minerals, complex carbohydrates, and fiber. Leafy greens provide high levels of calcium, phosphorus and other important minerals. Vegetables provide a feeling of light, clean eating. Eat at least two or three servings of vegetables per day to ensure optimal nutrition and healthful digestion.

Leafy Greens	*Round and Ground*	*Roots*
Asparagus	Artichokes	Burdock
Beet greens	Bamboo shoots	Carrots
Carrot tops	Beets	Celery
Chinese cabbage	Broccoli	Chicory root
Collard greens	Brussels sprouts	Daikon radish
Curly dock	Cabbage	Dandelion root
Daikon greens	Cucumber	Icicle radish
Dandelion greens	Green peas	Jinenjo
Endive	Leeks	Lotus root
Escarole	Mushrooms	Parsnip
Kale	Okra	Red radish
Kohlrabi	Squashes	Rutabaga
Lamb's quarters	Acorn squash	Salsify root
Leek greens	Butternut squash	Turnip
Lettuce	Hokkaido pumpkin	
Mustard greens	Hubbard squash	
Parsley	Pumpkin	
Plantain	Yellow squash	
Scallion	Zucchini	
Shepherd's purse	Snow peas	
Sorrel	String beans	
Sprouts	Sweet potatoes	
Swiss chard	Yams	
Turnip greens		
Watercress		

Cooking Vegetables

Steaming—Steam for 3 to 5 minutes, depending on their size and consistency, in a 1/2 inch of water.

Boiling—Boil in water with a couple of drops of tamari soy sauce for 3 to 5 minutes. Nutrients are lost in greater quantities when vegetables are boiled in a larger volume of water over a longer period of time. Reuse vegetable broth in soups and sauces to add nutrients.

Sautéing—Sauté with good quality oils (sesame is ideal). Lightly coat frying pan, add washed and cut vegetables, and sauté for about 5 minutes.

Baking—The best way to prepare squashes. Cut squash, bake at 375° to 400°F for 1 to 2 hours until tender. Summer squash and zucchini require far less time—20 to 35 minutes depending on size. Yams and sweet potatoes require higher heat, between 400° and 500°F for about 1 hour.

Beans

Beans provide high quality protein and carbohydrates. They are also delicious and provide a luscious addition to every meal.

Azuki	Soybeans, including yellow
Black-eyed peas	and black soybeans
Chick-peas	Split peas
Kidney beans	Black beans
Lima beans	*Tempeh*, *tofu*, and *natto*
Lentils	(a fermented soybean
Navy beans	product)
Pinto beans	

Cooking Beans

Boiling—The preferred method for cooking most beans. Soak beans overnight and boil them with a single stalk of kombu, which will cause the beans to be more digestible and contain more minerals. Add a pinch of sea salt or a few drops of tamari

soy sauce when the beans are 80 percent done. Boil for about
1 1/2 to 2 hours.

Pressure cooking—Be sure that pressure cooker regulator is
clear and clean before pressure cooking beans because beans can
clog the regulator and cause problems in cooking. Add 3 cups
of water per cup of beans; cook with a stalk of kombu. Cover
pressure cooker, lock shut, bring to pressure, as indicated by the
hissing of the regulator (usually requires approximately 10
minutes), reduce heat to low, and cook for 45 minutes.

Baking—Place beans in pot of water; 3 to 5 cups of water
per cup of beans; add stalk of kombu, if desired, and a pinch of
sea salt. Bake at 350°F for 3 to 4 hours. When beans are 80
percent done, add a variety of condiments or spices, such as
miso, tamari soy sauce, and others.

Try tempeh, tofu, and natto.   Tempeh and tofu can be fried,
baked, steamed, and boiled; they can be added to soups and
stews. Tofu can be eaten raw. Add fresh grated ginger and a drop
or two of tamari soy sauce to enhance the flavor.

Sea Vegetables

Sea vegetables, or seaweeds, are among the most nutritious foods
on the planet. About 3 ounces of *hijiki*, or 100 grams, contains
1,400 milligrams of calcium; the same quantity of *wakame* contains 1,300 milligrams of calcium. Hijiki also contains 56 milligrams of phosphorus, 29 milligrams of iron, and 150 international units of vitamin A, or beta-carotene. Sea vegetables
are rich in a rich variety of trace minerals, such as zinc, magnesium, and manganese. Many sea vegetables also contain sodium
alginate; studies have shown that sodium alginate binds with
radioactive nuclides and chemical pollutants, leaches them out
of bones and tissues, and helps eliminate them from the body
through the intestinal tract. In short, sea vegetables are among
the most healthful and important foods on the planet today.

Rinse and soak sea vegetables thoroughly before using to
remove excess sodium.

Alaria
Cut alaria into small pieces, boil or add to soups and stews;
cook for 30 minutes. Rich in B vitamins, vitamins C and K,
and many trace elements.

Arame
Cook arame for 30 minutes with carrots, onions, lemon juice,
alone or in soups and stews. Rich in vitamins A and B, carbohydrate, calcium, many other minerals, and trace elements.

Dulse
Rich in protein, vitamins A, C, E, and B vitamins, iodine,
minerals, and trace elements, dulse can be roasted and added to
rice and other grains as a condiment; or added to soups and
stews.

Hijiki
Hijiki is loaded with nutrition, including protein, vitamin A, and
B family, calcium, phosphorus, iron, and many trace elements.
Boil with carrots, onions, daikon radish, for 1 hour to 1 1/2
hours.

Irish moss
Irish moss is used as a thickening agent for soups and stews,
rich in vitamins A, B$_1$, iron, sodium, calcium, and other trace
elements.

Kombu
Use stalks of kombu when cooking beans to soften them and
make beans easier to digest. Cooked also as a vegetable with
carrots, onions, with rutabagas, turnips, and daikon. Rich in
many nutrients.

Nori
Nori is perhaps the easiest sea vegetable to use and the one most
acceptable to the novice pallate. Nori comes in sheets, used to
make nori rolls, *sushi*, and rice balls (brown rice covered with

nori). Roast nori over an open flame for 5 seconds; when it turns bright green, remove from flame. Nori can be crumpled into a condiment. Rich in vitamins A, B family, C, and D, calcium, phosphorus, iron, and trace elements.

Wakame
Wakame is a leafy, rich sea vegetable, used mostly in soups (miso soup) and stews. Cooks in 20 minutes. Very nutritious.

Miso Soup

Like tamari soy sauce, miso is a fermented soybean product that provides an abundance of friendly bacteria to assist in digestion and food assimilation. Antibiotics indiscriminately kill bacteria in the body, including intestinal flora which are essential to healthy digestion. Miso and other fermented foods help to promote good digestion by repopulating the intestinal tract with friendly bacteria.

Miso is a rich and delicious food that one can easily overdo. It does contain sodium, too much of which can cause a variety of illnesses, including high blood pressure, kidney disorders, and stomach cancer. Use miso carefully. Enjoy a variety of misos, but for daily use the lighter, younger misos, such as rice, barley, and millet misos are best. The darker misos, such as *Hatcho*• (soybean), should be used for medicinal purposes and under the guidance of a trained health counselor. Add about a quarter of a teaspoon per cup of soup. Miso soup provides a rich and delicious broth that can be eaten daily.

Cooking Miso Soup

Miso soup begins by adding wakame to boiling water. Simmer. Cut vegetables while the wakame cooks and then add vegetables and cook until vegetables are soft—usually about 20 minutes. Reduce flame to low. Add miso to broth, cook for a few minutes, and then serve hot.

Carrots and onions are standard vegetables in miso soup, along with wakame.

There are a wide variety of misos. Dark misos, such as Hatcho, are better used in winter, while the red and barley misos are used year-round.

Animal Foods

Eat fish before poultry and poultry before beef or other red meats. Fish is lower in fat than red meat and poultry. The white meat of poultry is lower in fat than the skin and dark meat, and much lower than most red meats. White-meat fish, such as haddock, cod, and flounder are low in fat and highly nutritious foods. Salmon contains the omega-3 polyunsaturated oils that have been shown to reduce blood cholesterol level.

Condiments and Dressings

Roasted sesame seeds provide an excellent condiment on grains and noodles. Roast the seeds in a dry frying pan and then grind them until they are dry flakes and broken seeds. Separate one batch of seeds to use as one type of condiment. To a second batch of roasted sesame seeds add roasted and ground-up kombu, which adds minerals and taste to the sesame seed condiment.

You can add roasted and ground-up dried sardines to a third batch of sesame seed condiment. The recipe is as follows: roast the seeds; roast the dried sardines; grind both the seeds and the fish together and then sprinkle on whole grains, vegetables, and noodles. This condiment, called *chirimen iriko* or *chuba iriko*, provides lots of vitamins, protein, and minerals, including calcium from the bones of the fish.

Other healthful condiments:

Rice vinegar	*Umeboshi* dressings
Tofu-based salad dressings	*Mirin*

146

Olive oil in small amounts
  on vegetables occasionally
Grated gingerroot
Lemon juice, sliced lemons,
  as on fish

Horseradish
Scallions, chives, parsley
Natural tamari soy sauce
Miso dressings

Snacks and Desserts

Use unrefined, natural foods as snacks. Avoid oily, salty, sugared, or processed foods. Use whole grains as snacks for their fiber, vitamin, and mineral content.

Rice cakes
Dried fruit in season
Cooked fruit in season
Popcorn
Puffed grains
Natural candies made without
  sugar

Use natural sweeteners,
  including sweet rice syrup,
  barley malt, and maple
  syrup in cooking
Amazaké, or sweet brown rice
  dessert, available in most
  natural foods stores

Bread

Good quality whole grain bread, preferrably sourdough. Steam bread before eating as much as possible. It is easier to digest after lightly steamed.

Use natural, unsweetened apple butters, jams, and other spreads. Avoid sugar, fat, and chemical additives in all jams and spreads. As much as possible, avoid tahini, peanut and sesame butters.

Where the Nutrients Are

Vitamins

Vitamin A
The vegetable in its vegetable form, called beta-carotene, has been shown to be a powerful cancer preventive. Studies have shown

that even cigarette smokers benefit from the preventive properties of beta-carotene. The type of vitamin A found in animal products, such as eggs, liver, and milk, has not been shown to be as effective a preventor of cancer and other illnesses as beta-carotene.

Vitamin A also prevents night blindness and promotes development of bone and teeth, healthy skin, hair, and mucous membranes.

Foods that are rich in vitamin A are all squashes, carrots, broccoli, collard greens, cantaloupe, apricots, prunes, peaches, and watermelon.

Vitamin B_1

Thiamine, or B_1, is essential in the metabolism of carbohydrates and the healthy functioning of the nervous system. Deficiencies of thiamine cause beriberi. Sources of this important vitamin include whole wheat, brown rice, and other whole grains; nuts, berries, soybeans, and sunflower seeds.

Vitamin B_2

Niacin assists in digestion and the utilization of carbohydrates in the cells. Deficiencies cause pellagra (which includes diarrhea, skin irritations, and rash). Sources include whole grains, dried beans, legumes, and nuts.

Vitamin B_6

B_6, or pyridoxine, assists in the metabolism and absorption of fats and proteins and also in the formation of red blood cells. It is essential in the healthy functioning of the nervous system. Sources include green vegetables, whole grains, nuts, potatoes, corn, avocados, legumes, green peppers.

Vitamin B_{12}

Cobalamin, or B_{12}, is essential in the formation of red blood cells and the function of the nervous system. B_{12} deficiencies, which can take up to a decade to manifest, cause pernicious anemia, chronic fatigue, poor appetite, memory loss, tingling fingers, dementia, and a variety of nervous system disorders. Sources of B_{12} include all animal products, including red meat, eggs, dairy, poultry, and fish. B_{12} is also present in sea vegetables and oats. Fermented foods, long thought to be excellent sources of B_{12} by virtue of the bacteria that cause fermentation, have been questioned of late as adequate sources of the vitamin. This has given rise to new concerns among strict vegetarians over their intake of B_{12} and possible deficiencies. Lactating mothers need more B_{12} in order to pass the vitamin on to their nursing infants, and consequently should consider eating regular quantities of animal proteins, such as fish. The addition of small but regular amounts of fish, or fish condiment (roasted sesame seeds and roasted dried sardines, ground up together and sprinkled on grains) can provide healthful quantities of B_{12}.

Pantothenic acid
Pantothenic acid, one of the B complex vitamins, assists metabolism of foods and the creation of hormones. Sources include leafy greens, whole grains, nuts, cabbage, cauliflower, and fruit.

Vitamin C
Ascorbic acid, or vitamin C, is essential in the formation of the body's connective tissue, or collagen; it strengthens immune function, and helps prevent cancer. Sources of C include leafy green vegetables, such as collard, broccoli, and kale, citrus fruits, sprouted beans, squash, cabbage, and sauerkraut.

Vitamin D
Vitamin D is essential to the body's ability to utilize calcium and phosphorus for the development of healthy bones, teeth, muscle and nervous system tissues. Deficiencies can cause rickets, kidney damage, lethargy, and loss of appetite. Vitamin D is a fat-soluble vitamin that can be stored in the body. Historically, the principle source of vitamin D has been the sun. The sun's ultraviolet rays mix with fat molecules beneath the surface of the skin to create vitamin D. Less than an hour a day of sunlight or two hours on a weekend is considered sufficient to obtain

adequate quantities of vitamin D. Lactating mothers should get regular sunlight in order to ensure that their babies are receiving adequate vitamin D. Other sources include fish and fish oils; fish obtain vitamin D by eating plankton. Milk and milk products have been fortified with synthetic vitamin D, but since the vitamin is readily available from non-dairy sources there is no need for it to be consumed in this way. Vitamin D can be toxic if taken in high doses; people should avoid supplementation.

Vitamin E
Essential for the healthy development of red blood cells, muscles, and other tissues, vitamin E has been shown to help prevent breast cancer caused by nitrosamines (carcinogens found in barbecued meats and hot dogs). Vitamin E also plays a role in the development of hormones. Sources include leafy green vegetables, whole grains, especially whole wheat, dried beans, safflower oil, and the germ of wheat.

Vitamin K
Vitamin K is essential in the clotting of blood and bone metabolism. Sources include leafy greens, cauliflower, peas, soybeans, and soybean products, such as tempeh and tofu.

Minerals

Minerals are non-living or inorganic substances that come from earth or rock. Minerals are essential for cell function and formation. Many minerals, especially zinc, selenium, calcium, and iron, are essential to optimal immune function. To ensure that you are getting optimal amounts of minerals, eat whole foods, such as whole grains, fresh vegetables, sea vegetables (a rich mine of vitamins and minerals). Also, do not peel vegetables such as carrots, turnips, rutabaga, and parsnips but simply wash them so that the outer skin remains on the food. Also, use a cast iron skillet in cooking; your foods will leach iron from the skillet. Below are a list of important minerals often missing in a diet of refined foods.

Calcium

Calcium is essential for healthy bones, teeth, muscles, connective tissues, and immune function. The World Health Organization maintains that the average daily requirement of calcium be 400 milligrams. The U.S. recommended daily allowance is now 1,000 milligrams.

Calcium is abundant in green vegetables, especially collard greens, mustard greens, and kale. In fact, green vegetables are as potent a source of calcium as milk products, and even more healthful in light of the fact that milk products contain so much fat, antibiotics, and steroids. A cup of cooked collard greens contains 188 milligrams of calcium; a cup of milk contains only 181 milligrams.

Sea vegetables, such as hijiki, arame, dulse, nori, and wakame, are loaded with calcium. One hundred grams of hijiki (about 3 and a half ounces) contains about 1,400 milligrams of calcium. The same volume of wakame contains 1,300 milligrams of calcium.

Other foods that contain significant quantities of calcium are: 100 grams of broccoli contain 130 milligrams; 100 grams of dandelion greens, 187 milligrams; 100 grams of mustard greens, 138 milligrams; 100 grams of turnip greens, 184 milligrams; 100 grams of parsley, 203 milligrams; 100 grams of watercress, 151 milligrams; 100 grams of almonds, 254 milligrams; 100 grams of sesame seeds, 1,160 milligrams.

Many fish, especially sardines that still have the bones, contain large quantities of calcium as well. Canned sardines contain anywhere from 300 to 437 milligrams of calcium.

Many people are correctly concerned about the presence of oxalic acid, which binds with calcium and prevents it from being absorbed by the body. Beet greens, rhubarb, sorrel, spinach, and Swiss chard contain high quantities of oxalic acid, which makes these vegetables fairly useless in their nutrient contents.

However, studies have shown that the small quantities of oxalate found in other green vegetables are lost in cooking. Therefore, most green vegetables—especially those listed above— are excellent sources of calcium.

Phosphorus
Essential for healthy bones, teeth, muscle formation and function, phosphorus is plentiful in beans, whole wheat and whole wheat flour, leafy greens, buckwheat, brown rice, and barley.

Magnesium
Magnesium is essential for healthy development of teeth, bones, and is found in whole wheat and other whole grains, leafy greens, soybeans and soybean products, lemons, nuts, peaches, and seeds.

Iodine
The thyroid gland depends on the presence of iodine in the diet. Sources of iodine include fish, sea vegetables, Swiss chard, mushrooms, turnip greens, citrus fruits, watercress, and pears.

Iron
Iron is utilized by the hemoglobin of the blood to transport oxygen to cells. Excellent sources include fish, poultry, and other animal products, sea vegetables, split peas, millet, chick-peas, black beans, prunes, raisins, apricots, wheat germ, and leafy greens. Excess iron has been linked to liver disease and cancer. Consequently, supplementation of iron can be harmful.

Potassium
Potassium is essential in a vast array of cellular material and functions. It is necessary in the healthy functioning of cells, nerves, and muscles. It is used in the creation of protoplasm and acts with sodium to conduct electrical impulses through nerve fibers. Potassium is leached out of cells when excess sodium is consumed, causing edema.

Zinc
Zinc is essential to healthy immune function, healthy skin, and proper functioning of the sexual organs. Zinc has been shown to promote white blood cell count and enhance the strength of the immune system. Infants with low zinc have shown a greater

average rate of infection than those whose zinc levels are normal. Excellent sources of zinc include seafood, whole wheat, bulgur, and seeds (such as sunflower and pumpkin seeds).

Sodium

Sodium is essential to healthy nerve and digestive and immune function. It is an essential mineral for life.

When we think of sodium, we usually think of sodium chloride, or common table salt, which is 40 percent sodium. Salt has become an addiction for many people, who cannot eat a bit of food before they laden it with salt. The average American gets anywhere from six to eighteen grams a day of salt, but the body only needs a half a gram per day of sodium, and this can come from the food itself. In other words, there is no need for salt to be added at the table. Excess salt intake leaches calcium from the body and can be a factor in the onset of osteoporosis. The principal source of excess sodium is processed food, especially canned foods, though far too much sodium often appears in boxed and jarred foods, as well. Because so many processed foods are eaten, sodium has become a major health problem and has been shown to cause high blood pressure, edema, and stomach cancer. Salt can have a devastating effect on health when it is coupled with fat. Fat and salt together speed the onset of high blood pressure, which leads to other illnesses, including heart attack and stroke.

Excess salt is a problem, one that we must be conscious of. Nevertheless, salt does play an important role in cooking, especially the preparation of whole grains, because it opens the fibrous part of the grain and makes the food more accessible and more digestible. Salt also helps alkalize the food and, in small amounts, aids digestion.

Use high quality sea salt, which does contain trace minerals, such as zinc and magnesium. Sodium is essential to life. Also, avoid using salt at the table. Restrict the use of salt, tamari soy sauce, and miso to cooking and use these foods wisely.

Chapter 9

30 Days: A Program
for Prevention and Recovery

Now that you know the foods that make up the macrobiotic diet and what it can do for you once you adopt it, you need a few tips to get you going, and some guidance to keep you going, which is what this chapter is all about.

Below is a program that can be followed for *30 Days*. Our program is actually a 10-day menu plan that can be repeated three times, taking you through a month of macrobiotic eating. We have provided suggestions for three meals per day, plus snacks and desserts. In the next chapter is a series of standard recipes. We urge you to use these recipes, but also to purchase one or more of the macrobiotic cookbooks recommended in the Further Reading List at the back of this book.

We call this book *30 Days* because, after following the diet for that short time, you will find, see, and feel a difference in your life. Among the changes you are likely to experience will be some weight loss, an increase in energy, a clearing of the skin and mind, and a general feeling of lightness and aliveness. You may also experience some symptoms of discharge, as we explained in the previous chapter. These can include some temporary headaches, especially if you are coming off coffee, strong spices, lots of sugar or animal foods. The headaches, if any, should pass within a few days. You might also have a short-lived rash or a few days of frequent urination (especially if you are used to drinking a lot more liquid than you will be drinking on the diet), but these are unlikely to last more than three days. As long as the intestines are functioning well and urination is steady, your normal elimination organs will be able to discharge excess waste efficiently. However, if these organs are not functioning as well, you may experience some of the symptoms explained above.

Before we begin with the actual menus, let us talk about shortcuts, variety in breakfast and lunches, and snacks that can be added during the course of the day.

Shortcuts

BREAKFAST

Leftover grain:
When you make a whole grain for dinner, make enough for another two meals, such as breakfast or lunch for the following day. When you use a leftover grain for breakfast, add water for the morning meal to make the grain wetter and more digestible. The morning meal always should be a little moist to make it easier to digest. Also, if health permits, small amounts of brown rice syrup, barley malt, raisins, cooked fruit or *gomashio* can be added to the grain.

Cook breakfast grain the night before:
Whenever possible, cook the breakfast grain during the evening before. Steel-cut oats can be boiled in 20 minutes; when concluded, cover pot and turn off flame. Let the oats sit in their own heat overnight; they will be ready for you in the morning. Simply add a small amount of water, reheat, and add one of the suggested toppings, if desired.

Steamed sourdough bread:
Occasionally, steamed sourdough bread can be eaten at breakfast; add chopped leafy greens or unsweetened apple butter. Whole grains are far more preferable than bread. The grain begins to decompose the minute it is milled for flour, thus losing nutrients. Bread can be difficult to digest at times and can cause mucus production, especially if it is not chewed well.

Boxed cereals:
Occasionally, if health permits, you can use boxed dry cereals, such as Crispy Brown Rice by Erewhon or some other natural,

puffed grain, which are available in natural food stores. These cereals should be made of whole grains and free of all sweeteners and artificial additives. Instead of milk, use a combination of *bancha* tea and apple juice. All dairy products, including skim milk, should be avoided. Soy milks should be minimized because they are a little higher in fats. (Soybeans contain about 30 percent of their total calories in fat, which is largely polyunsaturated.)

LUNCH

Use leftovers:
Whenever possible, use leftover grains and vegetables from dinner the night before.

Use tempeh and tofu for lunch:
Both tempeh and tofu can be used in a wide variety of ways. Tempeh can be steamed, boiled, or fried; it is easily transported in a lunch box; and it can be used to make sandwiches on sourdough bread. It can be added to greens and mixed with a small amount of sauerkraut to make a delicious side dish.

Tofu also has great versatility. Unlike tempeh, tofu can be eaten raw. Grate fresh ginger onto the tofu, and sprinkle a few drops of tamari soy sauce on. Tofu can be used in sandwiches, with greens, sauerkraut, mustard, or ginger and tamari soy sauce.

Make rice balls for lunch:
Use leftover grains, especially brown rice, to make rice balls for lunch. Use sushi nori, which is preroasted and ready to eat; you will also need umeboshi plums or paste; and cooked brown rice. Place an umeboshi plum or umeboshi paste within a handful of cooked rice. (Umeboshi is a pickled plum available in natural food stores.) Moisten hands. Shape a quantity of rice into a ball—about the size of a baseball or smaller. Moisten hands again and shape a sheet of nori around rice so that it covers the rice as much as possible; use a second sheet if necessary, to cover the rice entirely. Let the nori dry. Now you have a ball of rice

and sea vegetable, made all the more tasty by the presence of the umeboshi plum or paste. A rice ball can be made in less than five minutes.

DINNER

Cook quantities of food on weekends and a single night per week and reheat before serving:
You can cook several cups of grains, beans, sea vegetables, soup, or desserts on Sunday to take you through Monday, Tuesday, and Wednesday. You can cook another quantity of these same foods on, say, Wednesday or Thursday night to take you to the weekend. Be sure to reheat your food before serving. Reheating restores flavor and awakens the food's underlying qualities.

Steam vegetables:
Steaming requires between three and seven minutes, depending on the type and quantity of the vegetable. Steam greens, carrots, and other vegetables before dinner each night. Eat a wide variety of greens, and eat greens daily.

Try some of the quicker grains:
For a change, try some of the prepared grains made by natural food companies, such as tabbouli, grain burgers, and tempeh burgers. These should be considered a break from the norm, however. These are, after all, processed foods. Our staple foods should be whole, fresh, and unprocessed.

DESSERTS AND SNACKS

In addition to the desserts suggested below, try those suggested in the previous chapter, such as amazaké. If health permits, use air-puffed popcorn; add puffed cereals to amazaké to make it more crunchy; use rice cakes with natural, unsweetened jams. Use brown rice syrup, barley malt, and fruit juice as sweeteners. Make oatmeal cookies and other desserts mentioned below.

Reduce or avoid all salty snacks; if your cholesterol is already high, or if you suffer from high blood pressure or angina pectoris, you should avoid snacks that include salt and oil, such as corn or potato chips. Salt causes kidney disorders and edema that can lead to high blood pressure.

Eating in restaurants:
Actually, it is not as difficult as you might think to enjoy a healthful meal in a restaurant. Restaurant eating is a break from the norm and should not be considered a way to improve your health. On the other hand, being too rigid and stuck to a conceptual dietary program can also be detrimental to health and happiness. The best idea is to follow your heart, your intuition, and good sense; be flexible and enjoy going out occasionally.

Here are some general guidelines:

When in a restaurant, order carefully, clearly and be firm. Most chefs, waiters and waitresses can be helpful and obliging if you know what you want and are clear about your requests. Keep your order simple and specific. In essence, you are asking that your food be cooked without the sauces, butter, or oil. In a Chinese restaurant, ask that your food be cooked without monosodium glutamate, or MSG.

Order fish, vegetables, and salad.

Fish: Scrod, cod, flounder, haddock, halibut, and other white-meat fish. Request that the fish be broiled or steamed and that no butter or oil be added. Avoid fried, baked, breaded, or sautéed fish. Avoid casseroles, scampis, and anything with a dairy base.

Vegetables: Many restaurants are happy to provide lightly steamed or boiled vegetables without adding butter or oil.

Salad: The better restaurants provide dark green lettuce, which is richer in nutrients, especially calcium, than iceberg lettuce. You can bring your own homemade dressings or request lemon for salad. Avoid fatty, dairy-based dressings which contain saturated fats.

Condiments: Use high quality mustards, horseradish, sauerkraut, and pickles.

Dessert: Fresh fruit in season and/or unsweetened fruit juice.

Oriental restaurants:
Oriental restaurants, especially Chinese and Japanese restaurants, are nearly ubiquitous today. They provide grain (usually white rice, but sometimes brown, too), steamed vegetables, and some harmless sauces (some of which are made of white flour and water). They often provide healthful soups and fresh fruit desserts.

Natural food restaurants:
Many cities and larger towns offer natural food restaurants where you can eat cleanly prepared fish, whole grains, vegetables, and natural food desserts. For those who travel a lot, the book *Vegetarian Times' Guide to Natural Foods Restaurants in the U.S. and Canada*, published by Avery Publishing Group is a must. In addition to bookstores, the book is available through the publisher in Garden City Park, New York or by contacting *Vegetarian Times* magazine, in Chicago, Illinois.

30 Days: A Program You Can Live with

Recipes for all of these foods are provided in the following chapter. Below the program, we have also provided a shopping list and an inventory of kitchen equipment that will be helpful in preparing these foods.

Variety is an essential aspect to healthful eating. However, if a particular grain dish, breakfast, or lunch is easier for you to prepare and eat because of scheduling conflicts, do not be afraid to repeat foods when the menu plan calls for change. However, keep in mind that no one food will provide you with the full complement of nutrients that your body needs. Therefore, vary your main meals, especially dinner, and eat a wide assortment of foods from the list provided in Chapter 8.

This menu is for ten days; repeat the menu on the days suggested so that you complete a month on this program. After a full *30 Days* period, you will be sufficiently familiar with all the foods to choose for yourself.

In addition to the meals listed below, be sure to follow the simple guidelines we have been providing throughout the book. Those are as follows, and some additional ones that are important, are the following:

1. Chew your food fifty to seventy times per mouthful.
2. Walk daily, weather permitting.
3. Be active. Spend less time sitting and more time engaged in activities that need addressing or are fun.
4. Eat until you are 80 percent full. Do not overeat; leave yourself a little empty. This will give you more energy and a clearer head. You will not feel sleepy after your meal, but fresh and alive.
5. Sit down and be at peace before you eat. If you stand or jump up and down during a meal, you will suffer indigestion and fail to benefit from the good food you are consuming. In other words, you will ruin all the efforts you have made. Try not to eat when you are upset. Be calm whenever you sit down for your meal. If necessary, take a walk before dinner or lunch. Walking will reduce stress and allow you to concentrate on your food.
6. Be grateful for the quality of food that is coming to you from the universe. This is the healthiest and highest quality food available and it is coming to you from nature itself. Be grateful for the efforts made by the earth and by the human hands that have brought this food to you.
7. Learn to cook the food. The macrobiotic foods are as delicious as any on the planet. This is not a deprivation diet, but one that is richer in flavors and textures than the standard Western fare. In order for you to fully appreciate the taste and beauty of this food, you will have to learn to properly prepare the food. Give yourself time to do this and do not quit until you have fully mastered the art of healthful cooking. At that point, you will control your health and you will have the freedom to eat as you please.
8. Change your diet at a pace that is appropriate for you. Some people who want to use the macrobiotic diet as a means of healing will want to adopt the program more

rapidly than those who are in generally good health. Whatever your health status, commit to the program and do your best to follow it. Allow yourself the time to adjust to the new tastes and adapt to the pleasures of the macrobiotic cuisine.

9. Recommit. There is not a person alive who does not fall off the wagon occasionally. Do not indulge in harsh recriminations of yourself. Be gentle, understand why you desired some other foods—were you eating too much salt or grain and not enough vegetables or variety? In other words, learn from your mistakes and move on. Commit to the diet, and recommit.

Now for the program.

Days: 1, 11, and 21

BREAKFAST
Miso soup, with vegetables and wakame
Scrambled tofu (Cut up a block of tofu, add turmeric, scallions or onions, a few drops of tamari soy sauce, some other vegetables, if desired, and fry in a skillet that is lightly brushed with sesame oil.)
Grain coffee

LUNCH
Brown rice, pressure-cooked (p. 174)
Waldorf salad (p. 189)
Sautéed leafy greens
Bancha tea (p. 250)

DINNER
Mushroom-barley soup (p. 214)
White-meat fish (p. 235)
Boiled daikon radish, sliced up in coins, and cooked with a few drops of tamari soy sauce
Chinese-style sautéed vegetables (p. 196)

Coffee gelatin
Bancha tea

Days: 2, 12, 22

BREAKFAST
Leftover mushroom-barley (miso) soup
Breakfast porridge (p. 176), plain or with any of the following
topings: approximately one third to one half teaspoon of
rice syrup mixed into porridge; one third to one half
teaspoon barley malt; raisins; roasted sunflower seeds;
roasted sesame seeds; or crispy rice cereal
Bancha tea

LUNCH
Fried noodles (p. 183)
Salad, pressed (pp. 193 and 194)
Applesauce (p. 225)
Bancha tea

DINNER
Lentil-vegetable soup (p. 216)
Brown rice with azuki beans, pressure-cooked
Steamed kale
Arame with carrots and onions (p. 205)
Cooked fruit compote

Days: 3, 13, 23

BREAKFAST
Bulgur and oatmeal
Grain coffee

LUNCH
Brown rice and azuki beans, leftover, with nori (crushed
onto the rice, as a condiment, or as rice rolled in nori)
Leftover steamed kale from last night's dinner

Spring water or fruit juice

DINNER
Noodles in tamari soy sauce
Steamed collard greens
Kidney bean salad
Apple crisp
Bancha tea

Days: 4, 14, 24

BREAKFAST
Oatmeal, plain or with desired topping
Bancha tea

LUNCH
Pressure-cooked brown rice, with any of a variety of
condiments listed in Chapter 8; or rice balls, rice wrapped
in nori
Tempeh, fried in sesame oil, with sauerkraut
Salad with orange miso dressing

DINNER
Vegetable soup (p. 221)
Millet with cauliflower
Steamed collard greens
Oatmeal cookies
Bancha tea

Days: 5, 15, 25

BREAKFAST
Breakfast polenta
Bancha tea

LUNCH
Vegetable soup (p. 221)
Sandwich made of steamed sourdough bread, leaftover leafy

greens, with small amount of mustard or toasted sesame oil dressing

DINNER
Broiled fish (p. 235)
Brown rice with gomashio
Wakame-cucumber salad (p. 209)
Nishime vegetables (p. 190)
Tamari pickles
Applesauce (p. 225)

Days: 6, 16, 26

BREAKFAST
Breakfast porridge with toppings (p. 176)
Bancha tea

LUNCH
Brown rice with nori, as nori rolls or nori that is crushed into bits and used as a condiment
Leftover nishime vegetables
Bancha or *Mu* tea or water

DINNER
Chick-pea soup (p. 218)
Fried noodles (udon or soba) with either kombu pickles or ginger pickles (p. 183)
Baked squash
Daikon, kombu, and daikon greens (p. 191)
Steamed leafy greens (any of the following: kale, collard, mustard greens, etc.; p. 188)
Coffee gelatin

Days: 7, 17, 27

BREAKFAST
Miso-vegetable soup (p. 213)
Bulgur and oatmeal with topping if desired

Bancha tea

LUNCH
Leftover grain or noodles
Boiled greens (p. 188)
Bancha tea
Fruit

DINNER
Corn soup (p. 215)
Pressure-cooked brown rice (p. 174)
Hijiki with onions and lotus root (p. 207)
Chick-peas and vegetables (p. 201)
Steamed leafy greens (p. 188)
Amazaké pudding with apples or pears (p. 223)

Days: 8, 18, 28

BREAKFAST
Leftover corn soup
Steamed bread with jam (unsweetened apple butter or some
other natural, unsweetened jam)
Bancha tea

LUNCH
Fried Rice, fried in sesame oil (fry rice from last night's
dinner; p. 177))
Water-sautéed vegetables (p. 192)

DINNER
Azuki bean-vegetable soup (p. 216)
Udon or soba and broth (p. 184)
Pressed Salad (pp. 193 and 194)
Dried tofu with kombu and carrots (p. 202)
Kanten (p. 227)

Days: 9, 19, 29

BREAKFAST
Bulgur and oatmeal with variety of toppings
Grain coffee

LUNCH
Leftover noodles; or sandwich of greens on whole wheat
sourdough, steamed, with mustard
Fruit dessert

DINNER
Soybean stew (p. 218)
Rice balls with either umeboshi paste or plum within and
covered with sushi nori (p. 175)
Steamed leafy greens (p. 188)
Steamed carrots
Coffee gelatin dessert
Bancha tea

Days: 10, 20, 30

BREAKFAST
Polenta
Bancha tea

LUNCH
Bulgur salad (p. 185)
Burdock and carrots *kinpira* (p. 193)
Boiled greens

DINNER
Millet squash soup (p. 219)
Brown rice with *tekka* condiment
Steamed Chinese-style vegetables
Dried chestnuts and apples (p. 225)
Bancha tea

A Shopping List

Before you buy anything, look over the menu plan carefully
and the recipes to get acquainted with the foods you will need
for the program. You can look over Chapter 8 again if anything
looks particularly unfamiliar. But to start off, let us buy a sampl-
ing of the foods listed below, which will be helpful in getting
you going. We are going to make some suggestions on the
quantities of foods to buy, but you will have to adjust these
directions depending on the size of your family and the number
of people you will be cooking for.

Whole Grains:

Buy at least a pound of the following grains:

> Brown rice
> Bulgur
> Barley
> Millet
> Corn
> Oats, steel-cut or whole
> Cornmeal for polenta

Noodles:

Buy one or two packages of the following noodles:

> Whole wheat noodles; any shape or size will be fine. Whole
> wheat noodles are sometimes sold in bulk; half a pound
> usually is enough for four servings.
> Whole wheat udon; a single 8-ounce package contains
> enough noodles for 3 or 4 servings.
> Soba, or buckwheat noodles; a single 8-ounce package
> contains enough noodles for 3 or 4 servings.

Vegetables:

Buy a variety of vegetables, especially leafy greens, round, and roots. Be sure the vegetables are fresh and, whenever possible organically grown. The following list will assist you in purchasing the more important vegetables.

Collard greens
Kale
Mustard greens
Dark green lettuce
Chinese cabbage
Broccoli
Squash; whatever is available in the season
Cabbage
Onions
Carrots
Brussels sprouts
Cucumber
Turnips
Rutabagas
Scallions (1 bunch)
Mushrooms
Shiitake mushrooms
Chives (1 bunch)
Daikon radish
Gingerroot

Beans:

Buy at least one pound of the following beans; 2 cups of beans provides approximately four servings.

Azuki beans
Chick-peas
Lentils
Black beans

Kidney beans
Split peas
Tofu (1 package provides 2 or 3 servings)
Tempeh (1 package provides 3 or 4 small servings)

Sea vegetables:

Buy at least one package of the following sea vegetables.

Arame
Hijiki
Sushi nori (Use sushi nori initially; ıt requires no roasting
—non-sushi nori requires roasting over an open flame or
burner—and can be used to wrap rice and other grains
for a quick and tastey condiment.)
Wakame
Kombu

Animal Foods:

Buy any of the following fish; one pound of fish will usually
provide 3 or 4 small servings.

Sole
Flounder
Haddock
Halibut
Cod

Condiments and dressings:

Tamari soy sauce (Buy a single bottle of the "lite" tamari
that is low in sodium.)
Miso (Buy two or three different misos, preferrably the rice,
barley, and millet misos. Try other misos to see which
flavors you enjoy most.)

Sesame seeds; one pound of sesame seeds will provide more than enough roasted condiment for several weeks
Rice vinegar

Desserts and snacks:

Apples and other fruit
Applesauce, unsweetened
A variety of dried fruits
Sunflower and pumpkin seeds
Apple juice
Popcorn
Rice cakes
Puffed grain cereals
Brown rice syrup, 1 jar
Barley malt, 1 jar
Whole wheat pastry flour, one pound
Whole wheat flour, one pound
Kuzu, a thickening agent (also called kudzu) used to make gelatins
Agar-agar, another thickening agent, also used to make gelatins, often in combination with kanten

Oils:

Sesame oil
Corn oil
Safflower oil
Olive oil

Beverages:

Bancha or *kukicha* twig tea, noncaffeinated pleasant tasting tea. Boil twigs in water, pour through a strainer.
Grain coffee substitute
Spring water

Mu tea (bead-like berries that are boiled in water and
strained, to make a mild-tasting, settling tea)
Fruit juices
Spring water

Kitchen Equipment

You will need to review your kitchen equipment to make sure
you have everything you will need to cook healthful meals.
Below is a short list of the utensils that you may need.

• *A stainless steel pressure cooker.* Pressure cookers lock in
the food's nutrients during cooking. Unlike aluminum and
teflon coated pots, stainless steel does not chip or peel and,
consequently, will not release little particles into the cooking.
While there are a variety of stainless steel pressure cookers, you
might consider the Presto or Aeternum pots, the latter of which
is particularly safe because the pot top fits inside the pot by
inserting the pot top inside the pot and turning it to create
a snug fit. Pressure cookers are safe and easy to use. Accidents
are easily avoided by making sure the regulator on the pot top
is clean and clear of food particles. Also, make sure the pot top
fits snugly onto the pot itself. This will prevent pressure from
escaping from below the lid.

• *A cast iron skillet.* Cast iron skillets increase the iron in our
food by allowing the iron to be leached into the food itself.

• *Stainless steel sauce pans*, a variety of sizes to give you
versatility in cooking and cooking amounts

• *A cookie sheet*, medium size

• *Baking pans* for beans

• *A heat diffuser* to spread heat evenly throughout the bottom
of the pot

• *A colander*

• *A good vegetable knife*

• *A steamer* for vegetables and for steaming bread to make the
bread more digestible

• *A vegetable brush* for washing vegetables

- *A vegetable grater*
- *A bamboo tea strainer* to strain kukicha and Mu teas
- *Large glass jars* for string grains and noodles

Conclusion

We eat for many reasons. Among the most immediate reasons is for sensorial pleasure; another is for the feeling of satisfaction a good meal gives us. But more than any other reason, we eat to stay alive. We need food to go on living. But as we have seen, food can either support health and longevity, or it can bring about premature sickness and death. It all depends on the kinds of foods we choose to eat.

This book has been our attempt at helping you improve your food choices. We have tried to reveal the major causes of illness today. There are many causes of disease, especially those poisons that pollute our air, water, and soil. We do not wish to minimize these toxins, nor do we wish to diminish the efforts of those people who are working to clean up the environment. Their work is essential to the future health of our planet and the human race.

Nevertheless, when treated correctly, the body has an almost miraculous ability to ward off many of the most hideous toxins. It also has the capacity to overcome even those illnesses called "terminal." The human powers of regeneration should never be underestimated. And these powers are at their best when the body is properly nourished.

While there are many sources of ill health in our lives today —especially those in the environment—each of us has the most control over a single one: our daily food.

Macrobiotics is a powerful tool in the treatment of all our ills, physical, mental, and spiritual. But like all tools, its power is in its use. Do not hesitate to begin the diet just because you feel you cannot fully adopt it now. Do the best you can by doing as much as you can. And keep at it. Commit and recommit.

Remember, all tools require years of practice, which amounts to trial and error. There can be no perfect diet overnight; diet is an evolving process. It changes as we change. Allow yourself time to evolve on the macrobiotic diet. Come to know the foods of the earth, the way they grow, their nutritional, energetic, and healing properties. Use food for your pleasure, your medicine, and your means of longevity. Do not be dogmatic, nor overly relaxed. Be balanced in your approach to your diet.

Your daily food affects every aspect of your life—the amount of physical energy you possess, as well as your psychological equilibrium.

For those dealing with a serious illness, the macrobiotic diet can help you affect a miracle in your life. Use the diet wisely and seek out expert medical care and macrobiotic counseling. Do not use the diet imprudently or, dogmatically. Get help from a variety of healers and physicians.

We have tried to show what the body can do when properly nourished. Indeed, there are no limits.

Chapter 10

Cooking to Lower Cholestorol

The guidelines that follow are broad and flexible. The standard macrobiotic way of eating offers a wide range of foods and cooking methods to choose from. You can apply them when selecting the highest quality natural foods for yourself and your family.

These suggestions are especially for people living in a temperate climate. Modifications are required if you live in a tropical or subtropical climate, or a polar or semi-polar region. It is also necessary to adjust diet when traveling to one of these regions, and consider each person's individual needs and condition. For this reason, it is advisable to meet with a qualified macrobiotic teacher or participate in programs such as the Macrobiotic Way of Life Seminar or Macrobiotic Residential Seminar presented by the Kushi Institute in Massachusetts in order to receive personal guidance.

Whole Cereal Grains

Whole cereal grains are the staff of life and are an essential part of a way of eating to lower cholestorol. For people in temperate climates, they may comprise up to 50 to 60 percent of daily intake. Below is a list of the whole cereal grains and grain products that may be included:

Regular Use	Millet
Short grain brown rice	Corn
Medium grain brown rice (in	Whole oats
warmer areas or seasons)	Whole wheat berries
Barley	Buckwheat
Pearl barley (*hato mugi*)	Rye

174

Other traditionally used
whole grains

Occasional Use
Long grain brown rice
Sweet brown rice
Mochi (pounded sweet rice)
Cracked wheat (bulgur)
Steel-cut oats
Rolled oats
Corn grits
Cornmeal
Rye flakes
Couscous
Other traditionally used
whole grain products

*Occasional Use Flour
Products*
Whole wheat noodles
Udon (wheat) noodles
Somen (thin wheat) noodles
Soba (buckwheat) noodles
Unyeasted whole wheat
bread
Unyeasted whole rye bread
Fu
Seitan
Other whole grain flour
products that were
traditionally used

Basic Pressure-cooked Brown Rice

2 cups organic brown rice, washed
2½–3 cups water
pinch of sea salt per cup of grain

Wash rice and place in a pressure cooker. Add water and place
the cooker on a low flame for about 10 to 15 minutes. Add the
sea salt and place the cover on the cooker. Turn the flame to
high and let the pressure come up. Reduce the flame to medium-
low and place a metal flame deflector under the cooker. Let the
rice cook for 50 minutes. Remove the pressure cooker from the
flame and allow the pressure to come down naturally. Remove
the cover and allow the rice to sit for 4 to 5 minutes. Remove
the rice with a bamboo paddle and place in a wooden serving
bowl.

Boiled Brown Rice

2 cups organic brown rice, washed
4 cups water

pinch of sea salt per cup of grain

Place the rice, water, and sea salt in a heavy cooking pot, cover, and bring to a boil. Reduce the flame to medium-low and simmer for about 1 hour or until all the water has been absorbed. Remove and place in a wooden serving bowl.

Rice Balls

1 cup leftover brown rice
pinch of sea salt
$\frac{1}{2}$–1 umeboshi
$\frac{1}{2}$ sheet toasted nori, cut in half

Dampen your hands slightly in a small bowl of water with the pinch of sea salt in it. Place the leftover rice in your hands and form into a triangular shape by cupping your hands into a "V" and applying pressure to mold the rice. The triangle should be firmly packed. With your index finger, poke a hole into the center of the rice and insert the umeboshi plum. Then close the hole by packing the triangle firmly again. Place 1 square of the toasted nori on the side of the triangle and the other square on the other side. Pack the rice triangle again so that the nori sticks to it. You may occasionally need to dampen your hands with a very small amount of the salted water to prevent rice and nori from sticking to them. If there are uncovered spots on the triangle you can patch them by sticking small pieces of toasted nori on them until the triangle is completely covered with nori.

Homemade Sushi

Homemade sushi (made from brown rice and non-chemicalized ingredients and without raw fish) can be eaten frequently as a snack, at parties, or as a handy lunch item. Many types of sushi can be made, using a variety of ingredients. The following recipe is for a simple vegetable sushi:

brown rice, cooked
nori

carrots
pinch of sea salt
scallion leaves
umeboshi plum or paste

Step 1:   Roast one side of a sheet of nori over a flame until it turns green and place on a bamboo sushi mat. Wet both hands with water and spread cooked brown rice evenly on the sheet of nori. Leave about 1/2 to 1 inch of the top of the nori uncovered with rice and about 1/8 to 1/4 inch of the bottom uncovered.

Step 2:   Slice a carrot into lengthwise strips 8 to 10 inches long and about 1/4 inch thick. Place carrot strips in water with a pinch of sea salt. Boil for 2 to 3 minutes. The carrots should be slightly crisp. Remove and allow to cool. Separate the green leaf portion of several scallions from the roots, so that each strip is about 8 to 10 inches in length. Place carrot and scallion strips approximately 1/2 to 1 inch from the bottom of the sheet of nori. Then lightly spread 1/16 to 1/8 teaspoon of puréed umeboshi along the entire length of the carrot and scallion strips.

Step 3:   Roll up the rice and nori, using sushi mat, pressing the mat firmly against the rice and nori until it is completely rolled up into a round log shape. The vegetables should be centered in the roll. If they are not centered, they were most likely placed too far from the bottom edge of the nori and rice.

Step 4:   Wet a very sharp knife and slice the roll into rounds that are about 1/2 to 1 inch thick. The knife may need to be moistened after each slice. If this is not done, the knife may not slice properly and it may cause the nori to tear.

Step 5:   Arrange rounds on a platter with the cut side up, showing the rice and vegetables, or pack in a lunch box.

Breakfast Porridge

1 cup organic brown rice, washed
5 cups water
pinch of sea salt

Place all ingredients in a pressure cooker and cover. Bring to
pressure, reduce the flame to medium-low, and cook for 50 to
55 minutes. Serve with umeboshi and roasted nori strips or your
favorite condiment and scallions.

Porridge with Vegetables

3 cups leftover brown rice
½ cup daikon, cut into matchsticks
½ cup carrots, cut into matchsticks
¼ cup onions, diced
¼ cup daikon greens (or other hard leafy greens)
sea salt or miso

Place rice in cooking pot with water. Place on the flame and
bring to a boil. Reduce flame to medium-low, cover, and simmer
for about 30 minutes. Then add the chopped vegetables to the
rice. Cook until the vegetables become soft. Add the greens
toward the end of cooking so that they will retain their bright
color. Reduce flame to low and season with either sea salt or
miso to taste. Place into individual serving bowls.

Fried Rice

2 cups brown rice, cooked
1–2 Tbsp dark sesame oil
1 Tbsp scallion roots, minced
1 cup onions, diced
½ cup celery, diced
½ cup carrots, sliced in thin matchsticks
½ cup burdock, sliced in thin matchsticks
1–2 Tbsp water, if the rice is dry
tamari soy sauce or sea salt
1 Tbsp parsley or scallions, chopped, for garnish

Place dark sesame oil in a skillet and heat up. Add the scallion
roots and sauté 1 minute. Next, place the onions and celery in
the skillet and sauté 1 to 2 minutes. Add the carrots and burdock. Place the rice on top of the vegetables and if the rice is

dry add water. Cover the skillet and reduce the flame to low. Simmer for 15 to 20 minutes or until the vegetables are soft and the rice is warm. Just before the vegetables and rice are done, add the tamari soy sauce to taste or a small amount of sea salt for a mild salt taste. Add the chopped parsley or scallions, cover, and cook, another 2 to 3 minutes. Mix all ingredients together and serve hot.

Brown Rice with Barley

1 cup brown rice
$\frac{1}{4}$–$\frac{1}{2}$ cup barley
$1\frac{1}{4}$–$1\frac{1}{2}$ cups water per cup of grains
pinch of sea salt

Wash rice and barley separately. Place in a pressure cooker and mix. Smooth surface of grain evenly. Add water and sea salt and place the cover on the cooker. Place on the flame and allow pressure to come up. Reduce flame to low, place flame deflector under the pot, and cook for 50 minutes. Allow pressure to come down, remove cover, and place in a serving bowl.

Brown Rice with Millet

1 cup brown rice
$\frac{1}{4}$ cup millet
$1\frac{1}{4}$–$1\frac{1}{2}$ cups water per cup of grains
pinch of sea salt

Wash rice and millet separately. Place in a pressure cooker and add water and sea salt. Cook as in the above recipe. Place in a serving bowl.

Sweet Rice and Chestnuts

2 cups sweet brown rice
1 cup chestnuts
$3\frac{3}{4}$–$4\frac{1}{2}$ cups water
pinch of sea salt per cup of grain and chestnuts

Wash chestnuts and dry roast them in a skillet for several minutes. Stir constantly and keep the flame low to prevent burning. When through roasting the chestnuts, soak them with water to cover for about 10 minutes.

Wash rice and place in a pressure cooker. Add roasted chestnuts and fresh water. Place cooker on a low flame for 15 to 20 minutes. Add sea salt and cover. Turn flame to high and bring to pressure. When pressure is up, place a flame deflector under cooker, and reduce flame to medium-low. Pressure cook for 50 minutes. After this time, remove rice and chestnuts from flame and bring pressure down. Serve in a wooden bowl.

Brown Rice and Lotus Seeds

1 cup brown rice, washed
$\frac{1}{4}$ cup white or red lotus seeds, soaked 3–4 hours
$1\frac{1}{4}$–$1\frac{1}{2}$ cups water
pinch of sea salt

Place rice, lotus seeds, and water in a pressure cooker. Put on a low flame for 10 to 15 minutes. Add sea salt and cover. Turn flame to high and bring to pressure. Cook as for plain rice.

Gomoku

1 cup brown rice, dry-roasted
1 Tbsp dried lotus root, soaked $\frac{1}{2}$ hour
1 piece dried tofu, soaked 10 minutes in warm water, rinsed in cold water, and diced
3 shiitake mushrooms, soaked, stems removed, and diced
1 Tbsp dried daikon, soaked 3–5 minutes, rinsed, and sliced
1 strip kombu, 2 inches long, soaked and diced
$\frac{1}{4}$ cup seitan, cubed
$\frac{1}{4}$ cup carrots, diced
$\frac{1}{4}$ tsp scallion root, finely chopped
$1\frac{1}{2}$ cups water
chopped scallions for garnish

Add all ingredients to a pressure cooker and cook as for plain rice. Remove from flame, allow pressure to come down, and remove cover. Allow to sit 4 to 5 minutes. Remove and place in a serving bowl. Garnish with chopped scallions and serve.

As a variation, rice may also be cooked with diced vegetables, vegetable water, soaking water from kombu, wakame, or shiitake, with bancha tea, or other ingredients. When using bancha tea instead of plain water, add a couple of drops of tamari soy sauce to the bancha and rice as well as the correct proportion of sea salt. There are thousands of variations that can be used when cooking rice. Please use imagination to create delicious rice dishes throughout the year.

Black Soybean Rice

> **1 cup brown rice**
> **¼ cup Japanese black soybeans**
> **1¼–1½ cups water per cup of grain**
> **pinch of sea salt**

Wash Japanese black soybeans and roast in a dry skillet until the skins begin to crack. Wash rice and place in a pressure cooker together with black soybeans. Mix and smooth surface of rice and black soybeans. Add water and sea salt and cover. Place on a high flame and allow the pressure to come up. Reduce the flame to low and cook for 45 to 50 minutes. Remove from flame and allow pressure to come down. Place in a serving bowl.

Brown Rice and Wheat Berries

> **1 cup brown rice, washed**
> **¼ cup wheat berries, washed and dry-roasted until golden brown**
> **1½–1¾ cups water**
> **pinch of sea salt**

Place rice, wheat berries, and water in a pressure cooker. Place on a low flame for 10 to 15 minutes. Add sea salt and cover. Turn the flame to high and bring up to pressure. Reduce flame to medium-low and place a flame deflector under the cooker. Cook for 50 minutes. Remove from flame and allow pressure to

come down. Remove cover and let sit 4 to 5 minutes. Place rice
in a wooden serving bowl. Garnish and serve.

Brown Rice with Fresh Corn

2 cups brown rice
1 cup fresh corn
2½–3 cups water
pinch of sea salt per cup of grain

Remove corn from the cob. Wash rice and place in a pressure
cooker. Add corn, water, and sea salt, and mix corn in with rice.
Pressure cook as for plain brown rice. Serve cooked rice with
an attractive macrobiotic garnish.

Mochi (Pounded Sweet Rice)

Mochi is cooked sweet rice that has been pounded for about 30
to 40 minutes or more, with a wooden pestle, until it becomes
sticky. It is then dried for 2 to 3 days.

Mochi can be purchased prepackaged in most natural food
stores. To serve, cut into small squares and dry roast in a skillet
until slightly browned on both sides, and the mochi puff up
slightly.

Mochi may also be steamed, baked, broiled, pan-fried in oil,
deep-fried or added to soups and stews. Mochi may be eaten
with a variety of toppings, including tamari soy sauce, warm
brown rice syrup, or toasted soybean flour (*kinako*). Mochi can
also be dry-roasted or toasted and placed in miso soup.

Millet with Vegetables

2 cups millet, washed
2½–3 cups water
1 cup hard winter squash, cut in 1-inch chunks
½ cup carrots, sliced in chunks
¼ cup cabbage, sliced in 1-inch squares
pinch of sea salt per cup of millet

182

Place all ingredients in a pressure cooker, cover, and bring to pressure. Reduce the flame to medium-low and cook for about 15 to 20 minutes. Remove and allow the pressure to come down. Remove the cover and place the millet in a wooden serving bowl. Garnish and serve.

Buckwheat (Kasha)

1 cup buckwheat groats, washed
pinch of sea salt
2 cups boiling water

Dry roast the washed buckwheat for about 5 minutes, stirring constantly. Place the sea salt and buckwheat in boiling water. Cover and reduce the flame to medium-low. Simmer for 20 to 30 minutes or until the buckwheat is soft and all water has been absorbed. Remove and place in a serving bowl, garnish, and serve. Persons with skin conditions or those who have had surgery in the past two years are advised to temporarily avoid buckwheat or products that contain it such as soba noodles.

Arepa (Corn Cakes)

Before preparing the arepas, we must prepare a dough, called *masa*. First cook the corn as above but use 4 cups of corn and 8 to 10 cups of water. Then remove and allow the corn to cool completely. Place the cooked corn in a hand grinder (do not use a blender) and grind to a soft consistency. Knead the ground corn for 10 to 15 minutes by hand. You may add a little water for a doughy consistency. You now have masa or corn dough. This will yield about 1 1/2 to 2 pounds of masa.

$1\frac{1}{2}$ lbs corn dough (masa)
$\frac{1}{4}$ tsp sea salt
water
dark sesame oil

Crumble the dough and add sea salt. Knead the dough with a small amount of water until it becomes soft. Form the dough into 6 to 8 fist-sized balls. Brush a small amount of dark sesame oil in a cast iron skillet and heat up. Flatten the balls of dough into round cakes about 1/2 inch thick, and cook for 2 to 3 minutes on each side, or until a crust forms on the cakes. Next, bake the cakes in a 350°F oven for about 20 minutes, or until the cakes puff up. The arepas are done when they make a hollow, popping sound when tapped.

Fried Noodles

> 1 package (8 oz) udon or soba
> 6 cups water
> 1 Tbsp dark sesame oil
> $\frac{1}{2}$ cup onions, sliced in thin half-moons
> 1 cup cabbage, shredded
> $\frac{1}{2}$ cup carrots, sliced in thin matchsticks
> $\frac{1}{4}$ cup scallions, sliced
> tamari soy sauce

Place the water in a pot and bring to a boil. Add the udon or soba and stir once or twice to prevent them from sticking. Return to boil. Reduce the flame to medium-high and cook several minutes until the noodles are the same color inside as outside. If the inside or center of the noodles is white or lighter in color than the outside, then cook a little longer. When done, place the noodles in a strainer or colander, and rinse thoroughly under cold water to stop the cooking action and to prevent the noodles from sticking together in clumps. Set the noodles aside and allow to drain. They are now ready to use.

Brush dark sesame oil in a skillet and heat up. Add the onions and sauté 1 to 2 minutes. Layer the cabbage and carrots on top of the onions. Place the noodles on top of the vegetables, cover, and cook on a low flame for 5 to 7 minutes until the vegetables are tender and the noodles are hot. Add the scallions and a small amount of tamari soy sauce for a mild salt taste, cover, and continue to cook 1 to 2 minutes until the scallions are done. Mix and place in a serving bowl.

Noodles with Vegetable-Kuzu Sauce

1 package (8 oz) udon, cooked
2½ cups water
3 shiitake mushrooms, soaked, stems removed, and sliced
1 strip kombu, 3–4 inches long, soaked
½ cup onions, sliced in ¼-inch-thick wedges
½ cup carrots, sliced on a thin diagonal
¼ cup celery, sliced on a thin diagonal
1 cup tofu, cubed and pan-fried until golden
1 cup broccoli, sliced in small flowerettes
3 Tbsp kuzu, diluted in 3 Tbsp water
1½–2 Tbsp tamari soy sauce
grated ginger for garnish (optional)
sliced scallions for garnish

Place the water, shiitake, and kombu in a pot and bring to a
boil. Cover and simmer 4 to 5 minutes. Remove the kombu and
set aside for future use. Continue to cook the shiitake for another
5 to 7 minutes. Add the onions, carrots, celery, tofu, and broccoli. Cover, reduce the flame to medium, and simmer until the
vegetables are tender but still slightly crisp and brightly colored.
Reduce the flame to low and add the diluted kuzu, stirring
constantly to prevent lumping. When thick, add the tamari soy
sauce for a mild salt taste, and simmer 2 to 3 minutes. Place the
cooked noodles in individual serving bowls and pour the
vegetable-kuzu sauce over them. Garnish with a dab of fresh
grated ginger and a few sliced scallions, and serve hot.

Udon or Soba and Broth

1 package (8 oz) udon or soba
1 strip kombu, 3 inches long, soaked
2 dried shiitake mushrooms, soaked and sliced
4 cups water
2–3 Tbsp tamari soy sauce
sliced scallions for garnish
1 sheet toasted nori, cut in 1-inch squares

Cook noodles, wash, and drain. Place kombu and shiitake in a
pot and add water. Bring to a boil. Reduce the flame to medium-

low and simmer for about 10 minutes. Remove kombu. (Either slice the kombu into small pieces and add again to the soup or leave it out and use it in some other dish.) Reduce the flame to low. Add tamari soy sauce to taste and simmer for 3 to 5 minutes. Place noodles in the pot of broth to warm them up. Do not boil them. Serve immediately. Garnish with slices of shiitake, scallions, and 1-inch squares of nori.

Noodle water may be saved and used as a beverage, or as a soup stock. Slightly soured noodle water may be used as a starter for sourdough bread, as it helps unyeasted bread to rise.

For variety, vegetables such as cabbage, onions, squash, carrots, broccoli, kale, and others, may be added to the unseasoned broth water in various combinations and cooked until tender. Then season with tamari soy sauce or miso.

Bulgur Salad

2 cups bulgur, cooked
¼ cup parsley, minced
¼ cup onions, minced
½ cup carrots, minced (lightly boiled for 1 minute)
½ tsp sesame oil
½ Tbsp tamari soy sauce
1 tsp lemon juice

Toss bulgur with cooking chopsticks or fork to cool and make fluffy. Mix in vegetables. Heat sesame oil and blend in a suribachi with tamari soy sauce and lemon juice. Mix in with salad and let sit for about a half hour before serving.

Whole Oats

1 cup whole oats, washed
5–6 cups water
pinch of sea salt

Place the whole oats in a pot. Add water and sea salt. (For a different flavor, roast the oats until light gold.) Cover and bring to a boil. Reduce the flame and simmer on a low flame overnight or for several hours. Place a flame deflector under the pot to keep oats from burning. This makes a very good breakfast cereal. Occasionally, add a few raisins or barley malt before eating.

Soft Pearl Barley Cereal

> 1 cup pearl barley, soaked 6–8 hours
> 5 cups water (soaking water)
> ½ cup onions, diced
> 2 shiitake mushrooms, soaked, stems removed, and diced
> pinch of sea salt
> chopped scallions for garnish

Place the soaked pearl barley and soaking water in a pressure cooker. Add onions, shiitake, and sea salt. Cover and place on a high flame. Bring up to pressure, place a flame deflector under the cooker and reduce the flame to medium-low. Cook for 50 minutes. Remove from the flame and allow pressure to come down. Place in individual serving bowls and garnish with chopped scallions.

Whole Wheat Sourdough Bread

There are many types of unyeasted whole wheat sourdough breads available in most natural food stores for occasional enjoyment. Whole wheat bread can be eaten plain, with various natural spreads, occasionally toasted, or steamed (which makes it moister and easier to digest). Generally, bread is eaten less often than noodles, especially when it is toasted. Onion, squash, or sesame butter can be used as a spread on occasion.

Vegetables

Roughly one quarter to one third (25 to 35 percent) of each person's daily intake can include vegetables. Nature provides an incredible variety of local vegetables to choose from. Those recommended for regular use include:

Regular Use
Acorn squash
Bok choy
Broccoli
Brussels sprouts
Burdock
Butternut squash
Cabbage
Carrots
Carrot tops
Cauliflower
Chinese cabbage
Collard greens
Daikon
Daikon greens
Dandelion leaves
Dandelion roots
Hokkaido pumpkin
Hubbard squash
Jinenjo
Kale
Leeks
Lotus root
Mustard greens
Onion
Parsley
Parsnip
Pumpkin
Radish
Red cabbage
Rutabaga
Scallions
Turnip
Turnip greens
Watercress

Occasional Use
Celery
Chives
Coltsfoot
Cucumber
Endive
Escarole
Green beans
Green peas
Iceberg lettuce
Jerusalem artichoke
Kohlrabi
Lambsquarters
Mushrooms
Patty pan squash
Romaine lettuce
Salsify
Shiitake mushroom
Snap beans
Snow peas
Sprouts
Summer squash

Wax beans

Avoid (for optimum health)
Artichoke
Bamboo shoots
Beets
Curly dock
Eggplant
Fennel
Ferns
Ginseng
Green/Red pepper
New Zealand spinach
Okra
Plantain
Purslane
Potato
Shepherd's purse
Sorrel
Spinach
Sweet potato
Swiss chard
Tomato
Taro (albi) potato
Yams
Zucchini

Vegetables can be served in soups, or with grains, beans, or sea vegetables. They can also be used in making rice rolls (macrobiotic sushi), served with noodles or pasta, cooked with fish, or served alone. The cooking methods used for vegetables include boiling, steaming, pressing, sautéing (both waterless and with oil), and pickling. A variety of natural seasonings, including, miso, tamari soy sauce, sea salt, and brown rice or umeboshi vinegar are recommended. To ensure adequate variety in the selection of vegetables, it is recommended that three to five vegetable side dishes be eaten daily.

Steamed Greens

This particular dish may be eaten daily or often. To prepare take greens such as turnip, daikon, carrot tops, kale, parsley, watercress, collards, cabbage, Chinese cabbage, radish tops, and others. Wash and slice them and place in a steamer or in a small amount of boiling water. Cover and steam several minutes until tender but still bright green.

If you are steaming several types of vegetables, it is best to do each separately to ensure even, proper cooking. They may be mixed after cooking. Also, the stems of green vegetables are often harder than the leafy portion and are best steamed separately, or at least chopped very finely before steaming.

It is convenient to use steamer basket for this method of cooking and to take about 2 to 3 minutes for steaming, depending upon the quantity and thickness of the vegetables used.

You may save the water from steaming for use as a soup stock, or as a base for a vegetable sauce which can be thickened with kuzu and lightly seasoned with sea salt, tamari soy sauce, or puréed miso. Serve over the vegetables.

Boiled (Blanched) Kale or Other Greens

In Japanese, this style of cooking is called *ohitashi*. Wash the kale, and either leave whole or slice. Place 2 to 3 inches of water in a pot and bring to a boil. Place the kale in the water, cover, and boil 1 to 2 minutes, until deep green but slightly crisp. Remove, drain, and place in a serving bowl.

The kale may be served plain or with a sauce such as kuzu, tamari-ginger, or sesame-umeboshi dressing. You may also garnish with roasted sesame seeds or a little gomashio.

Other green vegetables can also be cooked this way. Boil for a very short time, until the vegetables are tender but still have a crisp texture and a deep, vibrant color. The cooking time depends upon the vegetables. For example, watercress takes only 35 to 40 seconds, while collard greens may take 1 to 2 minutes.

Boiled (Blanched) Salad

This dish can also be served daily or often. Many kinds of boiled salad can be prepared simply by varying the combination of vegetables or the type of dressing served with the salad. Boiled salad can be served with or without dressing. The following is an example of boiled salad:

> **water**
> **1 cup Chinese cabbage, washed and sliced on a diagonal**
> **$\frac{1}{4}$ cup carrots, sliced in matchsticks**
> **2 Tbsp celery, sliced on a thin diagonal**
> **1 cup watercress, washed and left whole**

Place 2 to 3 inches of water in a pot and bring to a boil. Place the Chinese cabbage in the pot, cover, and boil for 1 to 2 minutes, or until tender but still a little crisp. Remove, place in a strainer, and allow to drain and cool. Next, place the carrots in the boiling water, cover, and simmer for 1 minute or so. Remove, drain, and allow to cool. Next, do the celery and then watercress. After draining the watercress, you may slice it in 1-inch lengths. Place all the cooked vegetables in a serving bowl and mix. Serve plain or with a dressing.

When making boiled salad, it is best to cook each vegetable separately in the same water. Cook the vegetables with the mildest tastes first, such as onions, daikon, or Chinese cabbage. Then do the stronger tasting ones like celery, burdock, and watercress.

Waldorf Salad

> **$3\frac{1}{2}$ cups cabbage, shredded**
> **$\frac{1}{4}$ cup carrots, grated**
> **$\frac{1}{2}$ cup walnuts, roasted and chopped**
> **$\frac{1}{4}$ cup celery, sliced finely on a diagonal**

1 apple, cut into ¼-inch slices or chunks
¼ cup raisins

Mix all ingredients in a salad bowl. Add a natural dressing (see below) and mix. Cool before serving.

Natural Dressings

1. Purée 1 umeboshi plum or 1 teaspoon of umeboshi paste with 1/2 cup of water in a suribachi. (Chopped parsley, scallions, or roasted sesame seeds may also be blended in for variety.)
2. Dilute 1/2 teaspoon of barley miso in 1/2 cup of warm water and add 1/2 to 1 teaspoon of brown rice vinegar. Mix.
3. Dilute 1 teaspoon of tamari soy sauce with 1/2 cup of water and a small amount of chopped parsley. Mix.
4. Lightly sprinkle a desired macrobiotic condiment on the salad.

Nishime Vegetables

1 strip kombu, 4 inches long, washed, soaked, and cut into
   1-inch squares
water
1 cup daikon, sliced in 1-inch-thick rounds
¼ cup turnips, sliced in thick chunks
1 cup buttercup or butternut squash, or Hokkaido pumpkin,
   sliced in large chunks
½ cup carrots, sliced in chunks
¼ cup fresh lotus root, sliced in ½-inch-thick rounds
¼ cup burdock, sliced on a thick diagonal
1 cup cabbage, sliced in 2-inch-thick chunks
pinch of sea salt
tamari soy sauce

Place the kombu on the bottom of the pot and add about 1/2 inch of water. Layer the vegetables on top of the kombu in the following order: daikon, turnips, squash, carrots, lotus root, burdock, and cabbage. Add a pinch of sea salt, cover, and bring to a boil. Reduce the flame to low and simmer for 30 to 35 minutes or until the vegetables are soft and sweet. Add several drops of tamari soy sauce, cover, and simmer for another 5 minutes or so until almost all remaining liquid is gone. Mix the vegetables to evenly coat them with the sweet cooking liquid that remains. Place in a serving bowl.

Daikon, Kombu, and Daikon Greens

2 cups daikon, sliced in $\frac{1}{2}$-inch-thick rounds
1 strip kombu, 2–3 inches long, soaked and cubed
1 cup daikon greens, sliced
water
tamari soy sauce

Place the kombu in a pot and set the daikon rounds on top. Add about 1/2 to 1 inch of water, cover the pot, and bring to a boil. Reduce the flame to medium-low and simmer for 20 to 30 minutes or so until the daikon and kombu are soft and tender. Season with a small amount of tamari soy sauce. Then, place the greens on top of the daikon, cover, and simmer 2 to 3 minutes until the greens become tender but still bright green. Mix and serve.

Dried Daikon and Kombu

This dish can be eaten approximately 2 to 3 times per week; 1 cup per meal is usually sufficient. This style of cooking is known as a kind of *nitsuke* style.

$\frac{1}{2}$ cup dried daikon, rinsed, soaked 10 minutes, and sliced
1 strip kombu, 4 inches long, soaked and sliced in thin
  matchsticks
water
tamari soy sauce

Place the kombu in a heavy skillet or pot and add the dried daikon. Include enough kombu soaking water to half or three quarters cover the daikon. Cover, bring to a boil, and reduce the flame to medium-low. Simmer for 30 to 40 minutes until soft and sweet. Add a small amount of tamari soy sauce for a mild taste, cover, and continue to cook several minutes until all liquid is gone.

Sautéed Vegetables

> dark sesame oil
> ½ cup onions, sliced in thin half-moons
> ½ cup carrots, sliced in thin matchsticks
> ½ cup cabbage, shredded
> pinch of sea salt or tamari soy sauce
> water

Brush a small amount of dark sesame oil in a skillet and heat up. Add the onions and sauté 1 to 2 minutes. Place the carrots in the skillet and sauté 2 to 3 minutes. Add the cabbage and a pinch of sea salt and sauté 1 to 2 minutes. Place several drops of water in the skillet, cover, and reduce the flame to medium-low. Simmer 4 to 5 minutes or until tender but still slightly crisp and brightly colored. If you choose to season with tamari soy sauce instead of sea salt, add it at the end of cooking.

Water-sautéed Vegetables

> water
> ½ cup onions, sliced in thin half-moons
> ¼ cup celery, sliced on a thin diagonal
> ½ cup carrots, sliced in thin matchsticks
> ½ cup Chinese cabbage, sliced on a thin diagonal
> dark sesame oil
> tamari soy sauce

Place enough water in a skillet to just cover the bottom and heat up. Add the onions and sauté 1 to 2 minutes. Add the celery and sauté 1 to 2 minutes. Place the carrots in the skillet and sauté 2 to 3 minutes. Set the Chinese cabbage on top of the other vegetables. Add a few more drops of water, cover, and reduce the flame to medium-low. Simmer 3 to 4 minutes until tender but still crisp. Add a few drops of tamari soy sauce, cover, and simmer another 1 to 2 minutes. Remove the cover and cook off any remaining liquid.

Burdock and Carrot Kinpira

> 1 cup burdock, shaved
> 1 cup carrots, sliced in matchsticks
> dark sesame oil (optional)
> water
> tamari soy sauce

Place a small amount of dark sesame oil in a skillet and heat up. Add the burdock and sauté for 2 to 3 minutes. Set the carrots on top of the burdock. Do not mix. Add enough water to lightly cover the bottom of the skillet and bring to a boil. Cover and reduce the flame to medium-low. Cook several minutes until the vegetables are about 80 percent done. This may take 7 to 10 minutes. Add a few drops of tamari soy sauce, cover, and cook for several more minutes. Remove the cover and cook until all remaining liquid evaporates.

Pressed Salad No. 1

> 1 cup daikon, sliced in paper thin rounds and then thin
>   matchsticks
> $\frac{1}{2}$ cup carrots, sliced in paper thin rounds and then thin
>   matchsticks
> $\frac{1}{4}$ tsp sea salt
> 1–2 Tbsp brown rice vinegar
> 1 tsp black sesame seeds, roasted

Place daikon and carrots in a pickle press. Add the sea salt and brown rice vinegar. Mix thoroughly. Place the top on the press and tightly screw down. Let sit 1 hour. Remove and squeeze out excess liquid or, if too salty, rinse quickly under cold water. Place in a bowl and garnish with the roasted black sesame seeds.

Pressed Salad No. 2

> 2 cups lettuce, thinly sliced
> ¼ cup celery, sliced on a thin diagonal
> ½ cup cucumber, sliced in thin rounds
> ¼ cup onions, sliced in very thin rounds
> ¼ cup red radish, sliced in very thin rounds
> 2–3 Tbsp umeboshi vinegar

Place all ingredients in a bowl and mix well. Place in a pickle press or bowl and apply pressure. Let sit for 2 to 4 hours. Remove and squeeze out excess liquid. If too salty, rinse quickly under cold water, then squeeze out excess liquid.

Seitan Vegetable Stew

> 2 cups seitan, cooked
> 1 strip kombu, 3–4 inches long, soaked and cubed
> ½ cup celery, sliced on a thick diagonal
> ½ cup onions, sliced in thick wedges
> 1 cup carrots, sliced in chunks
> 1 cup Brussels sprouts, washed and sliced in half
> ¼ cup leeks, sliced on a thick diagonal
> ¼ cup burdock, sliced on a diagonal
> 4 cups water, or tamari-seasoned cooking water from seitan
> tamari soy sauce
> 4 Tbsp kuzu, diluted in 4–5 Tbsp water
> sliced scallions for garnish

Layer ingredients in the following order: kombu, celery, onions, carrots, Brussels sprouts, leeks, burdock, and seitan. Add the water and bring to a boil. Cover and reduce the flame to medium-low. Simmer until the vegetables are soft. Season with a small amount of tamari soy sauce for a mild salt taste and simmer for several more minutes. Add the diluted kuzu, stirring constantly to prevent lumping. When thick, reduce the flame to low and simmer for 2 to 3 minutes. Place in individual serving bowls, and garnish with sliced scallions.

Tempeh Cabbage Rolls

5–6 slices of tempeh, 3 inches by 2 inches
5–6 green Cabbage or Chinese cabbage leaves
1–1½ cups water
1 Tbsp tamari soy sauce
¼–½ tsp fresh grated ginger
5–6 strips *kampyo* (dried gourd strips for tying), soaked and
   cut into 8–10-inch lengths
2 strips kombu, 6–8 inches long, soaked
1–1½ tsp kuzu, diluted in 1 tsp water
scallion slices for garnish

If you are using Chinese cabbage leaves, remove leaves from
stem and place in a small amount of boiling water for 2 to 3
minutes. If you are using green head cabbage, leaves are often
difficult to remove. Simply steam the entire head of cabbage
several minutes until leaves can be easily removed. Remove
leaves and allow to cool slightly.

Slice tempeh and place in a saucepan. Add water to just cover
tempeh. Add a little tamari soy sauce to provide a mild salt
taste. Add about 1/2 teaspoon of grated ginger or 3 to 4 large
slices of fresh ginger. Bring to a boil, cover, and reduce the
flame to low. Simmer 15 to 20 minutes. Remove and drain.

Wrap each piece of tempeh up in a cabbage leaf. Tie a strip
of kampyo (dried gourd) around each cabbage roll or fasten the
cabbage leaf with a toothpick. Place kombu in the bottom of a
skillet and set cabbage rolls on top of kombu. Add enough
water to half cover cabbage rolls. Bring to a boil, cover, and
reduce the flame to low. Simmer 5 to 7 minutes if you want the
rolls to be slightly crisp and bright green. For older people, sick
persons, or children cook 10 to 15 minutes until cabbage rolls
are very soft and tender. Cooked a long time, they are very easy
to digest.

Remove cabbage rolls and place in a serving dish. Thicken
remaining cooking water with diluted kuzu, stirring constantly
to prevent lumping. Season with a little grated ginger and
tamari soy sauce to produce a mild salt taste. Pour this sauce

over the cabbage rolls. Garnish with a few scallion slices and serve.

Corn on the Cob with Umeboshi

4–5 ears of fresh sweet corn
4–5 umeboshi plums
4 cups water

Place water in a pot and bring to a boil. Remove the husks from the corn and wash the ears quickly with cold water. Place the sweet corn in the boiling water, cover, and reduce the flame to medium-low. Simmer 3 to 4 minutes. Remove and place on a serving platter or dish. Serve with umeboshi, which can be rubbed on the corn.

Sweet and Sour Seitan with Vegetables

2 cups seitan, cooked and sliced
1 cup burdock, sliced in chunks
1 cup apple juice
3 cups seitan-tamari cooking water
3–4 Tbsp kuzu, diluted in 3–4 Tbsp water
small amount of brown rice vinegar
¼ cup chopped scallions

Place seitan, burdock, apple juice, and seitan-tamari cooking water in a pot. Bring to a boil. Cover and reduce the flame to medium-low. Simmer 5 to 7 minutes until burdock is soft. Reduce flame to low and add diluted kuzu and a small amount of brown rice vinegar. Simmer 2 to 3 minutes. When done, place in a serving bowl and mix in chopped scallions. Serve hot.

Chinese-style Sautéed Vegetables

dark sesame oil
2 cups cabbage, finely sliced
1 cup celery, sliced on a diagonal
pinch of sea salt

Brush a small amount of dark sesame oil in a skillet and heat up. Add cabbage. Sauté 1 to 2 minutes on high flame, stirring constantly to prevent burning and to sauté evenly. Add celery and sauté 1 to 2 minutes. Keep flame high to keep vegetables crisp. Mix in a pinch of sea salt. Continue to sauté for a short time; the vegetables should remain crisp. Remove and place in a serving bowl. Serve.

Whole Onions and Miso with Parsley

5–6 medium-sized onions, peeled and left whole
1–1½ Tbsp puréed barley miso
2 Tbsp parsley, chopped
2 strips kombu, 6–8 inches long, soaked and sliced
2 cups water (approximately)

Make 6 to 8 shallow slices in each onion to create a sectional effect. If you slice too deeply, onions will fall apart. Slicing will cause the onions to open slightly while cooking.

Place the kombu in the bottom of a pot and set onions on top of it. Add water to half cover the onions. Place several dabs of puréed miso on top of each onion. Cover and bring to a boil. Reduce the flame to low and simmer until onions are soft and translucent. Remove onions and place in a serving dish. Pour remaining liquid, about 1 1/2 cups, over the onions. If too much liquid remains in the pot, thicken it with 1 1/2 to 2 teaspoons of kuzu, diluted in a little water. Pour kuzu sauce over the onions. Garnish with chopped parsley and serve.

Chinese Cabbage with Tamari-Lemon Sauce

4 cups Chinese cabbage, sliced on a diagonal
2–3 cups water
2–3 tsp fresh-squeezed lemon juice
2–3 Tbsp tamari soy sauce

Place about 1 1/2 inch of water in a pot and bring to a boil. Add Chinese cabbage. Cover and simmer 1 to 2 minutes, stirring occasionally to cook evenly until Chinese cabbage is bright

green and slightly crisp. Remove, drain, and place Chinese
cabbage in a serving dish.

Combine 2 to 3 teaspoons of lemon juice, 1/2 cup of water,
and 2 to 3 tablespoons of tamari soy sauce. Serve with Chinese
cabbage and pour a teaspoon or so over it before eating.

Beans and Bean Products

Beans and bean products may be eaten daily or often, so that
they comprise about 5 to 10 percent of daily intake. The following may be used in cooking:

Regular Use	Navy beans
Azuki beans	Pinto beans
Black soybeans	Soybeans
Chick-peas (garbanzo beans)	Split peas
Lentils (green)	Whole dried peas

Occasional Use	*Occasional Use Bean Products*
Black-eyed peas	Dried tofu
Black turtle beans	Fresh tofu
Great northern beans	Natto
Kidney beans	Tempeh
Mung beans	

Beans and bean products can be cooked in the following ways:
with kombu (about 10 percent); with carrots and onions
(about 20 percent); with acorn/butternut squash; with chestnuts
(about 20 to 30 percent); in soup with vegetables; and with
whole grains (about 10 to 15 percent beans).

Azuki Beans with Kombu and Squash

1 cup azuki beans, soaked 4–6 hours
1 strip kombu, 1–2 inches long, soaked and diced
1 cup hard winter squash, cubed (use acorn, buttercup,
butternut squash or Hokkaido pumpkin; carrots or parsnips
may be substituted if squash is not available)

water
sea salt

Place the kombu on the bottom of a pot. Set the squash on top. Place the azuki beans on top of the squash. Add water to just cover the squash. Bring to a boil, cover, and reduce the flame to low. Simmer until about 80 percent done. Season with 1/4 teaspoon of sea salt per cup of azuki beans, cover, and continue to cook another 15 to 20 minutes until soft and creamy.

Azuki Beans with Wheat Berries

1 cup azuki beans, soaked 6–8 hours
$\frac{1}{4}$ cup wheat berries, soaked 6–8 hours
1 strip kombu, 3–4 inches long
water (soaking water may be used)
$\frac{1}{8}$–$\frac{1}{4}$ tsp sea salt
chopped scallions for garnish

Place kombu on the bottom of a pot. Place azuki beans and wheat berries on top of the kombu. Add water to just cover. Bring to a boil, cover, and reduce the flame to medium-low. Simmer 1 1/2 to 2 hours or until 70 percent done, adding water, occasionally as needed, just to cover. Add sea salt and simmer, another 1/2 hour or so until soft. Remove, place in a serving bowl, garnish with chopped scallions, and serve.

Soybeans and Kombu

1 cup soybeans, soaked 6–8 hours in $2\frac{1}{2}$ cups water
1 strip kombu, 6 inches long, soaked and cubed
$2\frac{1}{2}$ cups water
tamari soy sauce

Drain off soaking water and place the kombu and soybeans in a pressure cooker. Add fresh water and boil for 15 minutes, skimming off any skins that float to the surface. Cover the pressure cooker and bring up to pressure. Reduce the flame to medium-low, and cook for approximately 50 minutes. Remove from the flame and allow the pressure to come down. Remove the cover, add a small amount of tamari soy sauce, and simmer uncovered for another 5 to 10 minutes. Remove, garnish, and serve.

Black Soybeans

Black soybeans are washed and soaked in a slightly different way than other beans because of their soft skins. To wash, first dampen a clean kitchen towel. Place the black soybeans in the towel and cover completely. Roll the bean filled towel back and forth several times to rub off dust and soil. Place the beans in a bowl, dampen the towel again, and repeat. This can be done 2 to 3 times until the beans are clean. After washing the beans, place them in a bowl. Add about 3 cups of water for each cup of beans and 1/4 teaspoon of sea salt. Soak the beans 6 to 8 hours or overnight. Place the beans in a pot, together with the salt-seasoned soaking water, and bring to a boil. Do not cover the beans. Reduce the flame to medium-low and simmer until the beans are about 90 percent done, which may take about 2 to 3 hours. During cooking you may need to add water occasionally but add only to just cover the beans each time. As the beans cook, a gray foam will rise to the surface. Skim off and discard. Repeat until the foam no longer appears. When the beans are about 90 percent done, add several drops of tamari soy sauce. (Do not mix with a spoon.) You may, however, gently shake the pot up and down 2 to 3 times to mix the beans and coat them with bean juice, which will make the skins a very shiny black color. Continue cooking until no liquid remains. Total cooking time varies from 3 to 3 1/2 hours.

Pinto Beans with Vegetables

1 cup pinto beans, soaked
1 strip kombu, 3–4 inches long, soaked and diced
$\frac{1}{2}$ cup onions, diced or cut in wedges
$\frac{1}{4}$ cup celery, sliced on thick diagonal
$\frac{1}{8}$ cup fresh sweet corn

¼ cup carrots, cut in chunks
water
⅛–¼ tsp sea salt
chopped scallions for garnish

Place kombu on the bottom of a pot. Layer onions, celery, corn, and carrots on top of the kombu. Place the soaked pinto beans on top of the vegetables. Add water to just cover the pinto beans. Bring to a boil. Cover and reduce the flame to medium-low. Simmer about 2 hours or until 70 to 80 percent done, season with sea salt and continue to cook until tender, which may take approximately 1/2 hour or so. Remove, garnish with chopped scallions, and serve.

Kidney Beans with Miso

1 cup kidney beans, soaked
1 strip kombu, 3–4 inches long, soaked and diced
water
1½–2 tsp puréed barley miso

Cook kidney beans as black soybeans. Season with miso the last 10 to 15 minutes of cooking. Instead of miso, sea salt may be used as a seasoning.

Chick-peas and Vegetables

1 cup chick-peas, soaked 6–8 hours or overnight
½ cup celery, sliced on a thick diagonal
1 cup carrots, sliced in chunks
1 strip kombu, 1–2 inches long, soaked and diced
water
sea salt, tamari soy sauce, or puréed barley miso

Place the kombu, celery, carrots, and chick-peas in a pot and add water to just cover. Prepare using either of the methods described above. When 80 percent done, season with sea salt, tamari soy sauce, or puréed barley miso. If boiling, chick-peas may take 3 to 4 hours.

Green Lentils with Onions and Kombu

1 cup green lentils
1 cup onions, sliced in thick wedges or diced
1 strip kombu, 2 inches long, soaked and diced
water
sea salt
chopped parsley for garnish

Place the kombu in a pot and set the onions on top. Add the lentils. Add enough water to just cover the lentils. Bring to a boil, reduce the flame to medium-low, and cover. Simmer about 35 minutes or until about 80 percent done. Occasionally, during cooking you may need to add small amounts of water as the lentils expand and absorb liquid. Each time add just enough water to cover the lentils. When the lentils are almost done, season with approximately 1/4 teaspoon of sea salt per cup of the lentils. Cover and simmer another 10 to 15 minutes.

Dried Tofu with Kombu and Carrots

$\frac{1}{2}$ cup dried tofu, soaked and cubed or sliced in rectangles
1 strip kombu, 2–3 inches long, soaked and sliced in very thin matchsticks
1 cup carrots, sliced in thick matchsticks
water
tamari soy sauce

Place the kombu in a pot. Add the dried tofu and carrots. Add enough water to just cover the dried tofu and bring to a boil. Reduce the flame to medium-low, cover, and simmer about 25 to 30 minutes or until the kombu is soft. Add several drops of tamari soy sauce, cover, and continue to cook for 3 to 5 minutes. Remove the cover and simmer until excess liquid is gone.

Scrambled Tofu

1 cake (1 lb) fresh tofu, drained
dark sesame oil
$\frac{1}{2}$ cup onions, diced

¼ **cup celery, sliced on a thin diagonal**
¼ **cup carrots, sliced in matchsticks**
¼ **cup burdock, sliced in matchsticks**
chopped scallions for garnish
tamari soy sauce

Brush a small amount of dark sesame oil in the bottom of a skillet and heat up. Add the onions and sauté 1 to 2 minutes. Next add the celery and sauté 1 to 2 minutes. Set the carrots and burdock on top of the celery and onions. Crumble the tofu and spread on top of the vegetables. Cover and bring to a boil. Reduce the flame to medium-low and simmer until the tofu is soft and fluffy and the vegetables are tender. Add a small amount of chopped scallions and several drops of tamari soy sauce. Cover and simmer another 2 to 3 minutes.

Scrambled Tofu and Corn

1 cake (1 lb) tofu
3 ears fresh sweet corn, removed from cob
dark sesame oil
tamari soy sauce
½ **cup scallions, chopped**

Lightly brush a skillet with dark sesame oil and sauté the corn for 2 to 3 minutes. With both hands, mash tofu into small pieces. Place the tofu on top of the corn and cover. Simmer several minutes until corn is done and the tofu is light and fluffy. Season with a small amount of tamari soy sauce (should not be brown or salty) and garnish with chopped scallions.

As a variation sauté onions, corn, carrots, and tofu, or onions, corn, cabbage, and tofu. As an option, season with a pinch of sea salt or a small amount of umeboshi vinegar instead of tamari soy sauce to keep the color of the tofu more white, or to create a different flavored tofu.

Pan-fried Tofu

4–5 slices of fresh tofu, ½ inch thick

dark sesame oil
tamari soy sauce
$\frac{1}{4}$–$\frac{1}{2}$ tsp fresh grated ginger (optional)
chopped scallions for garnish

Lightly oil a skillet and heat the oil. Place the tofu in the skillet. Add a couple drops of tamari soy sauce on top of each slice and squeeze a drop of ginger juice on each slice. Fry until golden (2 to 3 minutes). Turn over and fry on the other side until browned. Again add 1 to 2 drops of tamari soy sauce and ginger juice on top of each slice of tofu. Flip the slices over again and fry for several seconds. Remove, place on a serving platter, and garnish with chopped scallions.

These tofu slices may be eaten as is, used in preparing sandwiches, or sliced and added to nishime or even stews.

Small children do not usually like the taste of ginger as it is very strong. When preparing for children, this may be omitted.

Tempeh with Sauerkraut and Cabbage

1 cup tempeh, cubed
$\frac{1}{4}$ cup sauerkraut, chopped
1 cup green cabbage, shredded
small amount of sauerkraut juice
tamari soy sauce

Heat a skillet and add the tempeh cubes. Place a drop of tamari soy sauce on each cube and brown slightly. Add the sauerkraut and cabbage. Add enough sauerkraut juice or plain water to half cover the tempeh. Bring to a boil, cover, and reduce the flame to low. Simmer about 20 to 25 minutes. Remove the cover and cook off any remaining liquid.

Tempeh and Scallions

10 oz tempeh, cubed
1 bunch scallions, sliced
water
tamari soy sauce

Place the tempeh in a saucepan and add enough water to half cover the tempeh. Bring to a boil. Cover and reduce the flame to low. Simmer 20 to 25 minutes until almost all the liquid is gone. Add the scallions and tamari soy sauce, cover, and simmer 1 to 2 minutes. Remove the cover and cook off remaining liquid. Place in a serving bowl.

Sea Vegetables

Sea vegetables may be used daily in cooking. Side dishes can be made with arame or hijiki and included several times per week. Wakame and kombu can be used daily in miso and other soups, in vegetable and bean dishes, or as condiments. Toasted nori is also recommended for daily or regular use, while agar-agar can be used from time to time in making a natural jelled dessert known as *kanten*. Below is a list of the sea vegetables used in macrobiotic cooking.

Regular Use (*almost daily*)	*Occasional or Optional Use*
Arame	Agar-agar
Hijiki	Dulse
Kombu	Irish moss
Wakame	Mekabu
Toasted nori	Sea palm
	Other traditionally used sea vegetables

Arame with Carrots and Onions

1 oz dried arame, rinsed, drained, and allowed to sit 3–5 minutes
½ cup carrots, sliced in matchsticks
½ cup onions, sliced in thin half-moons
dark sesame oil
water
tamari soy sauce

Lightly brush dark sesame oil in a skillet and heat up. Place the onions in the skillet and sauté 1 to 2 minutes. Place the sliced

carrots on top of the onions. Slice the arame and set on top of
the carrots. Do not mix. Add enough water to just cover the
vegetables but do not the arame and a very small amount of
tamari soy sauce. Bring to a boil, reduce the flame to medium-
low, and cover. Simmer for about 35 to 40 minutes. Lightly
season with a few drops of tamari soy sauce for a mild salt taste.
Cover and cook another 5 to 7 minutes. Remove the cover and
continue to cook until almost all liquid is gone. Mix and cook
off remaining liquid. Garnish and serve.

Arame with Snow Peas and Tofu

2 cups arame (1¼ oz dry weight), rinsed, drained, and sliced
1 cup snow peas, stems removed and washed
1 cup pan-fried tofu strips, 2 inches long by ¼ inch wide
dark sesame oil
water
tamari soy sauce

Place a small amount of dark sesame oil in a skillet and heat up.
Add the arame and sauté 1 to 2 minutes. Place the tofu on top
of the arame. Do not stir. Add enough water to just cover the
arame. Cover and bring to a boil. Reduce the flame to medium-
low and simmer about 30 to 35 minutes. Season with a small
amount of tamari soy sauce, cover, and simmer another 5 to
10 minutes. Add the snow peas and cook 1 to 2 minutes until
bright green but still crispy. Remove the cover and cook off any
remaining liquid. Mix and serve.

Arame with Onions and Sweet Corn

2 cups arame
1 cup onions, sliced in half-moons
1 cup fresh corn, removed from cob
dark sesame oil
water
tamari soy sauce

Wash arame and place in a colander to drain. Do not soak it.

Heat a small amount of dark sesame oil in a skillet. Add onions and sauté 1 to 2 minutes, stirring to cook evenly. Add arame and just enough water to cover and bring to a boil. Reduce the flame to medium-low and simmer about 30 minutes or so. Add sweet corn, and if desired, season with a little tamari soy sauce. Simmer until all liquid is gone. Place in a serving bowl and serve.

Hijiki with Onions and Lotus Root

Depending on the texture or hardness of the hijiki, the cooking time may vary. Softer varieties of hijiki may only need to be cooked 30 to 40 minutes until soft, while harder varieties may require as much as 1 hour cooking time. Please adjust the cooking time depending on the variety of hijiki that is available to you.

> **1 oz hijiki, washed, soaked 3–5 minutes, and sliced**
> **$\frac{1}{2}$ cup onions, sliced in thin half-moons**
> **$\frac{1}{2}$ cup fresh lotus root, washed, halved, and thinly sliced**
> **dark sesame oil**
> **water**
> **tamari soy sauce**

Lightly brush dark sesame oil in a skillet and heat. Add the onions and sauté 1 to 2 minutes. Add the lotus root and sauté 1 to 2 minutes. Place the hijiki on top of the vegetables. Add enough water to cover the vegetables but not the hijiki. Bring to a boil, cover, and reduce the flame to medium-low. Simmer for 30 to 45 minutes depending on the texture or hardness of the hijiki. Season with a few drops of tamari soy sauce for a mild salt taste, cover, and continue to cook another 10 to 15 minutes. Remove the cover, mix, and simmer until all remaining liquid is gone. Garnish and serve.

Hijiki Salad with Tofu Dressing

> **1 oz hijiki ($1\frac{1}{2}$–2 cups)**
> **1 cake (16 oz) tofu**

water
1 cup carrots, halved lengthwise and sliced on a diagonal
$\frac{1}{2}$ cup celery, sliced on a diagonal
3 umeboshi plums
1 medium onion, chopped very fine or grated
2 Tbsp parsley, chopped

Soak hijiki 3 to 5 minutes and slice. Place hijiki and a small amount of water in a pot and bring to a boil. Reduce the flame to low, cover, and simmer 30 minutes or so. Remove hijiki and drain. Set aside to cool.

Place a small amount of water in a pot and bring to a boil. Place carrots in water, cover, and simmer 1 to 2 minutes. The boiled carrots should remain slightly crisp. Remove and drain carrots, reserving the cooking water. Set carrots aside to cool. Place celery in the same water you boiled the carrots in and simmer about 1 minute. Remove celery, drain, and allow to cool. Mix carrots and celery with cooked hijiki and set aside.

Remove pits and place umeboshi plums in a *suribachi*. Add chopped or grated onion and grind until umeboshi makes a smooth paste. Place tofu in suribachi with umeboshi paste and grind until smooth and creamy. Remove from suribachi and mix in chopped parsley. Place tofu dressing in a small serving bowl and garnish with a little parsley in the center.

Place the hijiki and vegetables in a serving bowl. You may place a tablespoon of tofu dressing on each portion of hijiki salad as it is served or you may mix all the dressing with the salad before serving.

Boiled Kombu with Burdock and Carrots

2 strips kombu, 6 inches long, soaked and cubed
1 cup burdock, sliced on thick diagonals
$1\frac{1}{2}$ cup carrots, sliced in chunks
water
tamari soy sauce

Place the kombu in the bottom of a pot. Add the burdock and carrots. Add enough water to half cover the vegetables. Bring to a boil, cover, and reduce the flame to medium-low. Simmer for 30 to 35 minutes or until the kombu and vegetables are soft and tender. Season with a few drops of tamari soy sauce, cover, and simmer another 5 to 10 minutes. Remove the cover and cook off all remaining liquid. Mix and serve.

Wakame, Onions, and Carrots

1 oz dried wakame, washed, soaked, and sliced
$\frac{1}{2}$ cup onions, sliced in thick wedges
$\frac{1}{2}$ cup carrots, sliced in chunks
water
tamari soy sauce

Place the onions, carrots, and wakame in a pot. Add enough water to half cover the vegetables. Bring to a boil, cover, and reduce the flame to medium-low. Simmer 25 to 30 minutes or until the vegetables are soft. Add a few drops of tamari soy sauce for a mild salt taste. Cover and simmer another 10 to 15 minutes.

Wakame-Cucumber Salad

2 cups wakame, washed, soaked 10 minutes, boiled 2 to 3
minutes, rinsed under cold water, drained, and sliced into
1-inch pieces
$\frac{1}{2}$ cucumber, washed, sliced into very thin rounds, soaked in
mild salt water, pressed about 30 minutes, rinsed, and
drained
brown rice or umeboshi vinegar

Arrange portions of wakame and cucumber in individual serving dishes. Pour 2 to 3 drops of brown rice or umeboshi vinegar on each dish of salad and serve.

Wakame with Sour Tofu Dressing

3 cups wakame, soaked and sliced
1 cake (16 oz) tofu, drained
water

3 umeboshi plums, pitted
¼ cup sliced scallions or chives

Place a small amount of water in a pot and add wakame. Bring
to a boil. Reduce the flame to low, cover, and simmer 3 to 5
minutes. Remove and place wakame in a serving dish.

In a suribachi, purée umeboshi to a smooth paste. Add tofu
and purée until smooth and creamy. You may also add a little
tamari soy sauce for a different flavor. Place tofu in a serving
dish and garnish with scallion slices or chives. To serve, place
a spoonful of tofu dressing on top of each serving of wakame.

Dulse Salad

¼ cup dulse, washed, soaked, and sliced into ½-inch pieces
1 cup Chinese cabbage, sliced finely and boiled less than
** a minute**
½ cup daikon, cut into matchsticks and boiled 1½ minutes
½ cup carrots, cut into matchsticks and boiled 1½ minutes
¼ cup onions, sliced in half-moons and boiled 1 minute

Mix dulse and vegetables in a salad bowl. Add a natural dressing
and mix. Cool before serving.

Toasted Nori

Nori, a light, thin sea vegetable that usually comes in dried
sheets, does not require washing or soaking but to increase its
digestibility, it can be dry-roasted. Take a sheet of nori from the
package and hold it so that the smooth, shiny side faces upward.
Turn the flame on your stove to medium and hold the nori
about 6 inches above it. Slowly rotate or move the nori above
the flame until it changes from purplish brown to green. You
may cut it into strips or squares for use as a garnish on soups,
stews, noodles or grains, or simply break off small pieces and
eat as a snack. Toasted nori can also be used in making rice
balls and sushi by wrapping cooked rice and other ingredients
inside it. Please see the section on cereal whole grains for recipes.

Watercress Sushi

> **2 bunches watercress, cooked, rinsed, and allowed to drain**
> **2 sheets nori, toasted**
> **4–6 *shiso* leaves (from umeboshi container), 4–5 inches long**
> **2 Tbsp sesame seeds, roasted**

With both hands, squeeze out excess water from the watercress. Place a sheet of nori on top of a bamboo sushi mat. Take half of the watercress and spread it evenly to cover the lower half of the sheet of nori closest to you.

Take 2 to 3 shiso leaves and lay them lengthwise across the center of the watercress, forming a straight line. Sprinkle 1 tablespoon of the sesame seeds on top of the shiso in a straight line.

Tightly roll up the nori and watercress in the sushi mat just as if making rice sushi. Before unrolling the sushi mat and removing the watercress cylinder, squeeze the mat gently to remove excess water.

Place the nori-covered watercress roll on a cutting board and quickly slice it in half. Slice each half, quickly, into 8 equal-sized pieces about 1 inch long. If the roll is not cut as soon as it is made it falls apart easily. There should now be 8 pieces of watercress sushi.

Repeat the process again until all the watercress and nori are used to make 16 pieces of sushi.

Boiled Sea Palm and Vegetables

> **2 cups sea palm, soaked and sliced**
> **1 cup carrots, cut into thick matchsticks**
> **½ cup onions, sliced in thick half-moons**
> **water**
> **tamari soy sauce**

Place the sea palm, carrots, and onions in a pot and add about 1/2 inch of water. Cover and bring to a boil. Reduce the flame to medium-low and simmer about 30 to 35 minutes or until the sea palm is tender. Season with a small amount of tamari soy sauce and simmer another 10 to 15 minutes until all remaining liquid is gone.

Vegetable Aspic

> **5–6 Tbsp agar-agar flakes (or read directions on package for appropriate amount)**
> **½ cup carrots, cut into matchsticks or flower shapes**
> **½ cup onions, sliced in thin half-moons**
> **½ cup celery, sliced on a thin diagonal**
> **1 quart water, kombu stock, or vegetable stock**
> **tamari soy sauce**
> **1 tsp ginger juice**

Blanch the carrots, onions, and celery separately for less than 1 minute, remove, and drain. Place the vegetables in a shallow casserole dish.

Place the water or stock in a pot and add the agar-agar flakes. Bring to a boil, stirring occasionally to dissolve the flakes, and then reduce the flame to low and simmer 2 to 3 minutes. Add a few drops of tamari soy sauce and the ginger juice. Mix and pour the hot liquid over the vegetables. Allow to sit in a cool place until jelled. Slice and serve.

As a variation, grated carrots or puréed squash can be used to make a delicious vegetable aspic.

Sweet azuki beans or split pea aspics are also very delicious.

Soup

Soups may comprise about 5 to 10 percent of each person's daily intake. For most people, that averages go out to about one or two cups or bowls of soup per day, depending on their desires and preferences. Soups can include vegetables, grains, beans, sea vegetables, noodles or other grain products, bean products like tofu, tempeh, or others, or occasionally, fish or seafood. Soups can be moderately seasoned with either miso, tamari soy sauce, sea salt, umeboshi plum or paste, or occasional ginger.

Light miso soup, with vegetables and sea vegetables, is recommended for daily consumption, on average one small bowl or cup per day. *Mugi* (barley) miso is recommended for regular consumption, followed by soybean (Hatcho) miso. A second bowl or cup of soup may also be enjoyed, preferably seasoned mildly with tamari soy sauce or sea salt. Other soup varieties include:

Bean and vegetable soups
Grain and vegetable soups (i.e., brown rice, millet, barley, pearl barley, etc.)
Puréed squash and other vegetable soups

Miso-Vegetable Soup

4–5 cups water
½ cup wakame, washed, soaked, and sliced
2 cups onions, sliced in thin half-moons
3–4 tsp puréed barley or soybean (Hatcho) miso
sliced scallions for garnish

Place the water in a pot and bring to a boil. Add the wakame, reduce the flame to medium-low, cover, and simmer for 3 to 4 minutes. Add the onions, cover, and simmer another 2 to 4 minutes until the onions and wakame are tender. Reduce the flame to very low, and add the puréed miso. Simmer another 2 to 3 minutes. Place in individual serving bowls and garnish with a few sliced scallions. Serve hot.

Kombu may be substituted for wakame. Simply soak for 3 to 4 minutes, slice in very thin matchsticks, and simmer for 5 to 10 minutes before adding the vegetables; or leave whole, simmer for 3 to 5 minutes, and remove.

Miso Soup with Rice

4–5 cups water
2 cups brown rice, cooked
¼ cup wakame or kombu, washed, soaked, and sliced
1 cup sliced scallion and scallion roots

3 tsp puréed barley or soybean (Hatcho) miso
sliced scallion for garnish

Place water in a pot and bring to a boil. Add the wakame or kombu, cover, and simmer for 3 to 4 minutes. Add the scallions, scallion roots, and cooked rice. Cover, reduce the flame to medium-low, and simmer about 10 minutes or so. Reduce the flame to very low and add the puréed miso. Cover and simmer 2 to 3 minutes. Place in individual serving bowls and garnish with sliced scallions.

Daikon-Shiitake Miso Soup

1 cup daikon, sliced in thin rounds, halved, or quartered
3 shiitake mushrooms, soaked, stems removed, and sliced
4–5 cups water
¼ cup wakame, soaked and sliced
1½–2½ Tbsp puréed barley (mugi) miso
sliced scallions for garnish

Bring the water to a boil and add the shiitake. Cover, reduce the flame to medium-low, and simmer 5 to 10 minutes. Add the wakame and simmer for 3 to 4 minutes. Place the daikon in the pot, cover, and simmer 2 to 3 minutes. Reduce the flame to very low, add puréed miso, cover, and simmer 2 to 3 minutes. Garnish with sliced scallions and serve.

Mushroom-Barley Soup

5 medium-sized shiitake mushrooms, soaked, stems removed, and
  sliced thin
½ cup barley
5–6 cups water
1 onion, diced
1 small carrot, diced
¼ tsp sea salt
1 stalk celery, diced
tamari soy sauce

Wash barley and place in a pot with water. Bring to a boil,

reduce the flame to low, cover, and simmer about 25 minutes. Add onions, shiitake, and carrots. Bring to a boil, reduce the flame, and simmer another 10 to 15 minutes. Add sea salt and celery and cook another 5 minutes. Season with tamari soy sauce to taste if necessary. Garnish and serve.

Barley-Lentil Soup

> ½ cup barley, washed and soaked
> ¼ cup lentils, washed
> 1 strip kombu, 4–5 inches long, soaked and diced
> ½ cup onions, diced
> 5–6 cups water
> ¼ cup celery, diced
> 5–7 fresh mushrooms, sliced
> ¼–½ tsp sea salt
> sliced scallions for garnish

Set the kombu on the bottom of a pot. Place the onions in the pot. Set the barley on top of the onions. Place the lentils on top of the barley. Add water. Bring to a boil, reduce the flame to medium-low, and simmer until the barley is almost done. Add the celery, mushrooms, and sea salt. Cook for another 15 to 20 minutes. Garnish with sliced scallions and serve.

For a variation, a combination of barley, kidney beans, onions, celery, and mushrooms is delicious.

Corn Soup

> 4 ears of fresh corn
> ¼ cup navy beans
> 1 stalk celery, diced
> 1 onion, diced
> 5–6 cups water
> ¼ tsp sea salt
> tamari soy sauce to taste if extra seasoning is desired

Wash navy beans and corn. Remove corn from ears with a knife. Place celery, onions, corn, and navy beans in a pot. Add water

216

and a pinch of sea salt. Bring to a boil, reduce the flame to low, cover, and simmer until navy beans are soft. Add remaining sea salt and a small amount of tamari soy sauce if necessary. Garnish and serve.

Azuki Bean-Vegetable Soup

1 cup azuki beans, washed and soaked 6–8 hours
1 strip kombu, 1 inch long, soaked and diced
½ cup onions, sliced
¼ cup celery, sliced on thick diagonals
1 cup butternut squash, cubed
¼ cup carrots, sliced in chunks
4–5 cups water (the azuki bean soaking water may be used as part of this measurement)
¼–½ tsp sea salt
tamari soy sauce (optional)
sliced scallions or chopped parsley for garnish

Place the kombu in a pot. Add the onions, celery, butternut squash, and carrots. Place the azuki beans on top. Add the water, cover, and bring to a boil. Reduce the flame to medium-low and simmer until about 80 percent done. Add the sea salt and continue to simmer until completely soft, which may take another 20 to 25 minutes. You may add several drops of tamari soy sauce just before serving for a slightly different flavor but it is not necessary. Garnish with sliced scallions or chopped parsley and serve.

Lentil-Vegetable Soup

1 cup green lentils, washed
1 strip kombu, 4–5 inches long, washed, soaked, and diced
½ cup onions, diced
¼ cup celery, diced
½ cup carrots, diced
2 Tbsp burdock, diced
4–5 cups water
¼–½ tsp sea salt

1 cup whole wheat elbow pasta, cooked, rinsed, and drained
¼ cup parsley, chopped
tamari soy sauce to taste (optional)

Place the kombu, onions, celery, carrots, and burdock in a pot.
Set the lentils on top. Cook as above. When 80 percent done,
add the sea salt and cook another 20 minutes. Add the cooked
whole wheat elbow pasta and the chopped parsley. Cook another
5 minutes or so. You may add a little tamari soy sauce for a
mild salt taste if desired, at the same time you add the pasta.

Kidney Bean Soup

2 cups kidney beans, soaked 6–8 hours
1 strip kombu, 3–4 inches long, soaked and diced
1 cup onions, diced
¼ cup celery, sliced on a diagonal
½ cup carrots, sliced in rounds
5–6 cups water
¼–½ tsp sea salt
chopped scallions for garnish

Place kombu, onions, celery, carrots, and kidney beans in a
pressure cooker. Add water, cover, and bring to pressure. Reduce
the flame to medium-low and cook about 1 hour. Remove and
allow pressure to come down. Remove cover and season with
sea salt. Simmer uncovered for another 10 to 15 minutes. Garnish
with chopped scallions and serve.

For a different, more rich flavor, season with a little puréed
miso instead of sea salt.

Black Bean Soup (Turtle Beans)

1 cup black beans
4–5 cups water
1 cup onions, diced
¼–½ tsp sea salt
chopped parsley or scallions for garnish

Place the black beans in a pressure cooker with water. Bring up to pressure. Reduce the flame to medium-low and cook for 45 to 50 minutes. Allow pressure to come down. Remove the cover and add the onions and sea salt. Simmer for another 20 minutes until the onions are soft. If desired, add a little tamari soy sauce to taste. Garnish with chopped parsley or scallions and serve.

Chick-pea Soup

    1 cup chick-peas, soaked 6–8 hours
    1 strip kombu, 3–4 inches long, soaked
    $\frac{1}{8}$ cup burdock, quartered
    $\frac{1}{2}$ cup onions, diced
    $\frac{1}{2}$ cup carrots, diced
    $\frac{1}{4}$ cup celery, diced
    4–5 cups water
    $1\frac{1}{2}$–$2\frac{1}{2}$ tsp puréed miso
    chopped scallions or parsley for garnish

Place kombu chick-peas, vegetables, and water in a pressure cooker. Cover and bring up to pressure. Reduce the flame to medium-low and pressure cook for 1 to 1 1/2 hours. Allow the pressure to come down. Remove the cover, season with miso and cook for several minutes longer on a very low flame. Garnish with chopped scallions or parsley and serve.

Soybean Stew

    1 cup white soybeans, washed and soaked 6–8 hours
    1 strip kombu, 3–4 inches long, washed, soaked, and diced
    3 cups water
    2 shiitake mushrooms, soaked, stems removed, and diced
    $\frac{1}{4}$ cup dried daikon, washed, soaked, and sliced
    $\frac{1}{4}$ cup dried tofu, soaked and cubed
    $\frac{1}{4}$ cup celery, diced
    $\frac{1}{2}$ cup carrots, diced
    2 Tbsp burdock, diced
    3 Tbsp fresh or dried lotus root, soaked
    $\frac{1}{2}$ cup seitan, cooked
    tamari soy sauce to taste

grated ginger for garnish
sliced scallions for garnish

Place the kombu in a pressure cooker. Add the white soybeans
and water. Cover and bring up to pressure. Reduce the flame to
medium-low and cook for 30 minutes. Remove from the flame
and allow the pressure to come down. Remove the cover and add
the shiitake, dried daikon, dried tofu, celery, carrots, burdock,
lotus root, and seitan. Place the cover back on the pressure
cooker and bring up to pressure again. Reduce the flame to
medium-low and simmer another 20 to 25 minutes. Remove
from the flame and allow the pressure to come down. Remove
the cover, add a small amount of tamari soy sauce for a mild
salt taste, and simmer another 3 to 4 minutes. Place in individual
serving bowls and garnish with a dab of grated ginger and a few
sliced scallions.

Millet Squash Soup

$\frac{1}{2}$ **cup millet, washed and dry-roasted until golden yellow**
1 cup winter squash, cubed
1 strip kombu, 1 inch long, soaked and diced
$\frac{1}{4}$ **cup celery, diced**
$\frac{1}{2}$ **cup onions, diced**
$\frac{1}{4}$ **cup dried daikon, soaked and sliced**
$\frac{1}{4}$–$\frac{1}{2}$ **tsp sea salt**
4–5 cups water
sliced scallions for garnish
toasted nori strips for garnish

Layer the ingredients in a pot in the following order: kombu,
celery, onions, dried daikon, winter squash, and finally millet
on top of the vegetables. Add a small pinch of sea salt and
enough water to just cover the millet. Cover and bring to a boil.
Reduce the flame to low and simmer until the millet is soft.
This may take about 30 minutes. Occasionally, during cooking,
you may need to add water, as the millet expands and absorbs
water. Add only enough to just cover the millet each time until
the millet is done. When done, you may add a little more water

for the desired thickness you choose and add the remaining sea salt. Cover and continue to cook another 10 minutes or so. Place in individual serving bowls, garnish with sliced scallions and toasted nori strips, and serve.

Puréed Squash Soup

**4 cups buttercup squash or Hokkaido pumpkin, washed, skin
and seeds removed, and cubed**
¼–½ tsp sea salt
4–5 cups water
sliced scallions or chopped parsley for garnish
toasted nori strips for garnish

Place the buttercup squash or Hokkaido pumpkin in a pot and add a small pinch of sea salt and the water. Cover and bring to a boil. Reduce the flame to medium-low and simmer several minutes until the squash is soft. Remove the squash and purée in a hand food mill to a creamy consistency. Place back in the pot, season with sea salt, and continue to cook another 10 minutes or so. Place in serving bowls, garnish with sliced scallions or chopped parsley and toasted nori strips, and serve.

French Onion Soup

2 cups onions, sliced in very thin half-moons
**1 strip kombu, 3–4 inches long, soaked and sliced in
matchsticks**
3–4 shiitake mushrooms, soaked and sliced
4–5 cups water
dark sesame oil
pinch of sea salt
2–3 Tbsp tamari soy sauce
¼ cup deep-fried whole wheat bread cubes
sliced scallions for garnish

In a pot, place kombu and shiitake and add 4 to 5 cups of water including the soaking water from the kombu and shiitake. Cover and bring to a boil. Reduce the flame to medium-low and simmer 3 to 4 minutes. Sauté the onions in a small amount of

dark sesame oil for about 5 minutes. Add the onions to the
water and add a pinch of sea salt. Simmer 25 to 30 minutes.
Add the tamari soy sauce and simmer another 10 minutes.
Garnish with deep-fried whole wheat bread cubes and sliced
scallions and serve.

Vegetable Soup

$\frac{1}{2}$ cup leeks, sliced in 1-inch pieces
1 cup onions, cut in thick wedges
$\frac{1}{2}$ cup celery, sliced on a thick diagonal
1 cup carrots, cut in irregular shapes
$\frac{1}{4}$ cup burdock, sliced diagonally
dark sesame oil
1 strip kombu, 3–4 inches long, soaked and cut into 1-inch cubes
$\frac{1}{2}$ cup dried tofu, soaked and cubed
4–5 cups water
pinch of sea salt
1–2 Tbsp tamari soy sauce
sliced scallions for garnish

Sauté the leeks and onions in a small amount of dark sesame
oil. Place the kombu, leeks, onions, celery, dried tofu, carrots,
and burdock in a pressure cooker. Add water and a pinch of
sea salt. Cover and bring to pressure. Cook for 10 to 15 minutes.
Allow the pressure to come down and remove the cover. Season
with tamari soy sauce and simmer for another 10 minutes.
Garnish with sliced scallions and serve.

This soup may be boiled for 45 to 60 minutes instead of
pressure cooking.

Cream of Corn Soup

2 ears fresh sweet corn removed from the cob
4 cups water
sesame oil
1 cup onions, diced
$\frac{1}{4}$–$\frac{1}{2}$ tsp sea salt
$\frac{1}{4}$–$\frac{1}{2}$ cup corn flour

¼ cup celery, diced
chopped scallions, parsley, or a sprig of watercress for garnish

Boil the corncobs in 4 cups of water. Save the water for the soup. Brush a pot with a very small amount of sesame oil. Sauté the onions and sweet corn. Add a pinch of sea salt. Add the corn flour to the onions and sweet corn. Mix so that the vegetables become coated with the flour.

Add the water, gradually, to the flour and vegetables, stirring gently but constantly to avoid lumping of the flour. Bring to a boil, reduce the flame to medium-low, and simmer about 30 minutes. Add the celery and remaining sea salt. Cook another 15 to 20 minutes. Garnish with chopped scallions, parsley, or sprig of watercress.

As a variation, omit the corn flour and season with tamari soy sauce instead of sea salt.

Fruit and Desserts

In general, fruit can be enjoyed on occasion by those in normal good health. Frequency of consumption varies according to climate, season, age, level of activity, and personal need and health considerations. The average is about two to four times per week.

Among fruits, locally grown or temperate climate varieties are preferred, especially for persons living in these regions. As much as possible, it is best to avoid consumption of tropical fruit. Below, the varieties of fruit that can be eaten in a temperate climate are presented according to season of availability or optimum season for use:

Spring	*Summer*	Grapes
Plums	Apricots	Peaches
Cherries	Blueberries	Raisins
Strawberries	Blackberries	Raspberries
Dried fruit	Cantaloupes	Strawberries
	Cherries	Tangerines
	Dried fruit	Watermelon

Autumn	Dried fruit	Prunes
Apples		
Pears	Dried Fruit (un-	Avoid in a Temperate
Grapes	sulfured)	Climate
Dried fruit	Apples	Banana
Raisins	Apricot	Dates
Apples	Peaches	Figs
	Pears	Pineapple
Winter	Raisins	Other tropical fruits
Pears	Cherries	
Raisins	Plums	

Stewed Fruit with Kuzu

1 cup apples or pears, sliced
1 Tbsp raisins
2 cups apple juice or water (or half and half)
pinch of sea salt
3 heaping tsp kuzu

Place the apples, raisins, apple juice or water, and a pinch of sea salt in a pot and bring to a boil. Reduce the flame to medium-low, cover, and simmer until the apples are soft. Turn the flame down low. Dilute the kuzu in a small amount of water and pour it into the apple mixture, stirring constantly to prevent lumping. When thick, simmer 1 minute. Remove and serve.

Amazaké Pudding with Apples or Pears

1 pint amazaké
1 cup apples or pears
3 tsp kuzu, diluted

Place the apples and amazaké in a saucepan and bring to a boil. Reduce the flame to medium-low and simmer until the apples are soft. Reduce the flame to low, add the diluted kuzu, stirring constantly to prevent lumping. Simmer 1 minute or so until thick. Remove and serve.

Cool Amazaké Cherry Pudding

1 quart fresh amazaké
pinch of sea salt
¼–⅓ cup kuzu
⅛–¼ cup water
1 cup cherries, pitted and sliced

Place amazaké and a pinch of sea salt in a saucepan. Dilute kuzu with a little water and add to amazaké. Bring to a boil, stirring constantly to prevent kuzu from burning and lumping. Once amazaké has thickened, simmer 2 to 3 minutes on a low flame. Mix in cherries. Place servings of pudding in individual serving dishes and set aside to cool. Instead of using individual serving dishes, you may simply place pudding in a bowl and let individuals serve themselves.

Stewed Plums

12 plums, halved (5½–6 cups)
3 cups water
½ cup raisins
pinch of sea salt
¼ cup barley malt
4 Tbsp kuzu
¼ cup almonds, slivered and roasted slightly

Wash plums, slice in half, and remove pits. Place water, raisins, sea salt, barley malt, and plums in a saucepan. Bring to a boil. Cover and reduce the flame to medium-low. Simmer about 7 to 10 minutes. Dilute kuzu with about 8 tablespoons of water and add it to fruit mixture, stirring constantly to prevent burning. Simmer until kuzu is translucent. Remove and place in individual serving dishes. Garnish each bowl with several slivered almonds. Serve.

Baked Apples

Wash the apples, core, and place in a baking dish with a little water. Cover and bake at 350° to 375°F for about 30 minutes or until soft. Remove and serve.

Baked Apples with Kuzu-Raisin Sauce

5–6 apples
1 cup apple juice
$\frac{1}{4}$ cup raisins
pinch of sea salt
1 Tbsp kuzu
1 Tbsp water

Place apple juice, raisins, and sea salt in a saucepan and bring to a boil. Reduce the flame to low and simmer, covered, for about 5 minutes. Dilute kuzu in water and add to apple juice and raisins. Stir constantly to prevent lumping. Set aside.

Wash apples (do not peel them) and bake in a baking dish with a little water at 375°F for about 15 to 20 minutes. To serve, place 1 apple in each individual serving bowl and spoon the kuzu-raisin sauce on top. Serve hot.

Applesauce

Wash, peel if waxed, core, and slice the apples. Place in a pot with a pinch of sea salt. Add enough water to just lightly cover the bottom of the pot. Cover and bring to a boil. Reduce the flame to medium-low and simmer until the apples are soft. Purée in a hand food mill. Serve.

Dried Chestnuts and Apples

1 cup dried chestnuts
$\frac{1}{2}$ cup dried apples, soaked and sliced
$2\frac{1}{2}$ cups water
pinch of sea salt

Wash the chestnuts and dry roast in a skillet, over a low flame for several minutes. Remove and place in a pressure cooker. Add the water and allow the chestnuts to soak for about 10 minutes. Add the dried apples and a pinch of sea salt. Place the cover on the pressure cooker and bring up to pressure. Reduce the flame to medium-low and simmer for about 40 minutes. Remove the cooker and allow the pressure to come down. Take the cover off and serve.

Azuki Beans with Chestnuts and Raisins

$\frac{1}{2}$ cup azuki beans, soaked 6–8 hours
$\frac{1}{2}$ cup dried chestnuts, dry-roasted and soaked 10 minutes
2 Tbsp raisins
1 strip kombu, 2–3 inches long, soaked and diced
$2\frac{1}{2}$ cups water
$\frac{1}{4}$ tsp sea salt

Place the kombu, azuki beans, chestnuts, raisins, and water in a pot. Cover and bring to a boil. Reduce the flame to medium-low and simmer for about 2 to 2 1/2 hours. As the azuki beans are cooking, you may need to add a small amount of water from time to time. When the azuki beans are about 80 percent done, season with sea salt, cover, and simmer for another 15 minutes or until soft.

Azuki, Chestnuts, and Raisin Compote

1 cup azuki beans, soaked 6–8 hours
1 cup dried chestnuts, washed, dry-roasted for 5–7 minutes,
    and then soaked about 10–15 minutes
$\frac{1}{2}$–$\frac{3}{4}$ cup raisins
1 strip kombu, 6–8 inches long, soaked and sliced in 1-inch squares
water
$\frac{1}{8}$–$\frac{1}{4}$ tsp sea salt

Place the kombu in a pot. Add chestnuts, raisins, and azuki beans. Add just enough water to cover azuki beans. Bring to a boil. Cover and reduce the flame to medium-low. Simmer about 2 to 2 1/2 hours. If necessary during this time, add water in small amounts only to just cover azuki beans. After 2 to 2 1/2 hours, season with a little sea salt. Continue to cook azuki beans until most of the remaining liquid has cooked away. Place in individual serving dishes and serve.

This dessert is especially delicious served over hot, fresh mochi.

Rice Pudding

2 cups brown rice, cooked
2 cups sweet brown rice, cooked
2 cups dried chestnuts
1 cup almonds, chopped
1 cup raisins
¼ tsp cinnamon (optional)
3½–4 cups apple juice

Dry roast the chestnuts in a skillet several minutes, stirring constantly to prevent burning. Remove chestnuts and soak covered with water for 10 to 15 minutes.

Place all ingredients including chestnuts in a pressure cooker and bring to pressure. Cook for 50 minutes. Remove from flame and bring pressure down. Remove cover and place pudding in a serving bowl. Serve hot.

Kanten

agar-agar flakes (follow package instructions for proper
amount of liquid)
4 cups water
pinch of sea salt
2 cups dried apples, soaked and sliced

Place the water, sea salt, dried apples, and agar-agar flakes in a pot. Bring to a boil, reduce the flame to low, cover, and simmer until the apples are soft. Remove and pour the apples and liquid into a dish. Refrigerate or place in a cool place until jelled. Kanten is usually ready to serve in 45 to 60 minutes. Slice or spoon into serving dishes.

Blueberry Pie

1 quart fresh blueberries

2–3 Tbsp water
pinch of sea salt
2–3 Tbsp yinnie (rice) syrup
2½–3 Tbsp kuzu

Wash blueberries and remove any stems or leaves. Place blueberries and water in a saucepan. Add a pinch of sea salt and bring to a boil. Reduce the flame to low, cover, and simmer about 2 to 3 minutes. Mix in yinnie syrup. Dilute kuzu in 2 1/2 to 3 tablespoons of water and mix in with the blueberries. Stir well to prevent lumping. Cook a few minutes until thick. Allow to cool slightly before placing in pie shell.

Pie Dough

4 cups wheat pastry flour
¼ tsp sea salt
⅛–¼ cup corn or sesame oil
¾–1 cup cold water

Mix flour and sea salt together. Add oil to the flour and mix it in well by sifting it with your hands. Add water and form flour into a ball of dough. Knead dough for about 2 to 3 minutes. Let it sit for about 5 to 10 minutes before rolling it out. Then divide dough in half and roll one part of it out.

Press half the dough into a pie plate to form the bottom crust and then add blueberries. Moisten outside lip of bottom crust with a little water to help seal the two crusts together once top crust is added. Roll out top crust and place on pie. With a wet fork, press edges down to seal the two crusts together. Poke several small holes in top crust with a fork. Place pie in oven and bake at 375°F for about 35 to 40 minutes or until crust is golden brown. Allow to cool before slicing.

Fruit Salad

½ cup honeydew melon, cubed
½ cup cantaloupe, cubed
½ cup watermelon, shaped in balls with a melon ball scoop

½ cup apples, sliced
lettuce leaves
pinch of sea salt

Place a few fresh green lettuce leaves in the bottom of a bowl. Mix the cut fruit and place it in the bowl on top of the lettuce leaves. Sprinkle with a pinch of sea salt, mix, and allow to sit about 15 minutes or so before serving.

Peach Crunch

Filling:
  10–12 peaches, washed and sliced
  pinch of sea salt
  1 cup water
  2 Tbsp kuzu
Topping:
  1 cup rolled oats
  ¼ cup walnuts
  ½ cup almonds
  ¼ cup sunflower seeds, washed
  2 Tbsp yinnie (rice) syrup or barley malt

Place peach slices, sea salt, and water in a saucepan. Bring to a boil. Cover and reduce the flame to low. Simmer about 5 minutes or until peaches are soft. Dilute kuzu in 2 tablespoons of water and add to the peaches, stirring constantly to prevent lumping. Simmer 2 to 3 minutes or until kuzu is translucent and thick. Place peaches in a baking dish.

For topping, lightly roast oats in a dry skillet on a low flame until golden brown. Stir constantly to prevent burning. Place roasted oats in a mixing bowl. Then lightly roast walnuts, almonds, and sunflower seeds separately in a dry skillet. Chop walnuts and almonds. Add walnuts, almonds, and sunflower seeds to oats. Mix yinnie syrup in well with oat-nut mixture. Sprinkle crunch over peaches.

Place peach crunch in a 350°F oven for about 15 to 20 minutes or until golden brown. Remove from oven and allow to cool slightly. Serve.

Macro Jacks

- **1 cup popcorn**
- **sea salt**
- **½ cup barley malt**
- **½ cup yinnie (rice) syrup**
- **2 cups peanuts, shelled and roasted**

Pop popcorn and season lightly with sea salt. Place barley malt and yinnie syrup in a saucepan and bring to a boil. Reduce the flame to low and simmer 3 to 4 minutes. Pour hot sweetener over popcorn and mix in well. Add peanuts and mix again. Place sweetened popcorn on an unoiled cookie sheet, making sure not to spread popcorn too thick on the sheet or it will not heat up properly. Bake at 350°F for about 10 minutes or until the syrup becomes darker and starts to bubble. Remove popcorn from the oven and allow it to cool. Baking causes the sweetener to harden on the popcorn. Place cooled Macro-Jacks in a bowl and serve.

Nuts

Nuts can be eaten from time to time as snacks and garnishes. In order to help lower cholesterol, it is best to keep their consumption occasional and to eat them in small amounts. Nuts are roasted and lightly salted (with natural sea salt) or a small amount of tamari soy sauce are preferred. Among the many types of nuts, non-tropical varieties that are lower in fat are recommended. Below are several varieties of nuts for use:

Occasional Use	*Nuts to Avoid (Tropical Varieties) for Optimum Health*
Almonds	
Peanuts	
Walnuts	
Pecans	Brazil nuts
	Cashews
	Hazel nuts
	Macadamia nuts
	Pistachio nuts

Roasted Nuts

Nuts can be roasted in two basic ways:

- *In the oven*—Place the nuts on a baking sheet and bake in a 350°F oven until slightly brown. When they are almost done, add a few drops of tamari soy sauce and mix to evenly coat. Bake another 2 to 3 minutes.
- *In a skillet*—Place a skillet on the stove and heat up. Add the nuts and reduce the flame to low. Stir constantly to evenly roast and prevent burning. Roast until light golden brown, sprinkle a few drops of tamari soy sauce on them and roast for another minute or two. Remove and serve.

Seeds

A variety of seeds may be eaten from time to time as snacks. They can be lightly roasted with or without salt. Varieties of seeds include:

Pumpkin seeds
Sesame seeds
Sunflower seeds
Other traditionally consumed seeds

Roasted Pumpkin or Squash Seeds

Rinse the seeds under cold water and drain. Heat a skillet and place the damp seeds in it. Dry roast, stirring constantly until the seeds become golden brown and begin to puff up slightly and pop. Plain roasted, unseasoned pumpkin or squash seeds are preferred, although on occasion you may season mildly with a few drops of tamari soy sauce, mix, and roast for another several seconds until the tamari soy sauce on the seeds becomes dry. Remove and place in a serving bowl.

Snacks

A variety of natural, high quality snacks can be eaten from time
to time. They can be made from grains, beans, nuts or seeds,
sea vegetables, and temperate climate fruits. The following foods
can be used as snacks:

> Leftovers
> Noodles
> Popcorn (homemade and unbuttered)
> Puffed whole cereal grains
> Rice balls
> Rice cakes
> Seeds
> Homemade sushi (without sugar, seasoning, or MSG)
> Mochi (pounded, steamed sweet brown rice)
> Steamed sourdough bread

Steamed Sourdough Bread

Slice several pieces of whole wheat sourdough or any other
unyeasted whole grain bread. Place about 1/2 inch of water in
a pot. Insert a steamer basket and place the sliced bread in the
steamer. Cover and bring the water to a boil. Reduce the flame
to medium and steam 4 to 5 minutes or until the bread is soft
and warm. Remove and serve as is, with miso-tahini spread,
naturally processed and salted sesame butter, or appropriate
spreads.

Miso-Tahini Spread

> **2–3 Tbsp organic sesame tahini**
> **barley miso**
> **1–2 Tbsp scallions, chopped**
> **water**

Place the tahini in a small saucepan. Add a small amount of
barley (mugi) miso for a mild salt taste, together with the

chopped scallions. Add several drops of water and mix well. Place on a medium flame and simmer 2 to 3 minutes until the scallions are cooked, mixing constantly to evenly cook and to prevent burning. Remove and serve on steamed bread, rice cake, or other appropriate snacks.

Sweets

The naturally sweet flavor of cooked vegetables is preferred for optimum health. One or several of the vegetables listed below can be included in dishes on a daily basis:

Cabbage	Parsnips
Carrots	Pumpkin
Daikon	Squash
Onions	

In addition, a small amount of concentrated sweeteners made from whole cereal garins may be included when craved. Dried chestnuts, which also impart a sweet flavor, may also be included on occasion, along with occasional consumption of hot apple juice or cider. Additional sweeteners include:

Amazaké (fermented sweet rice drink)
Barley malt
Brown rice syrup
Chestnuts (cooked)
Hot apple cider (with a pinch of sea salt)
Hot apple juice (with a pinch of sea salt)
Mirin (fermented sweet brown rice liquid)

Amazaké

Amazaké can be used in making desserts and puddings or may simply be heated in a saucepan and used as an occasional beverage.

Barley Malt or Brown Rice Syrup

These sweeteners may be used occasionally in making desserts, added in small amounts to soft cooked breakfast cereals, for a sweeter flavor, or added to bancha tea for an additional sweet flavor.

Chestnuts

(Please refer to the sections on whole cereal grains and desserts for recipes.)

Supplementary Foods

A variety of supplementary foods can be enjoyed occasionally in the standard macrobiotic diet. Some items can be eaten several times per week and others—such as seasonings and beverages—are used daily but in smaller amounts than the foods listed above. Supplementary foods include:

Fish

For variety, enjoyment, and nourishment, fish and seafood may be enjoyed on occasion by those in ordinary good health. The frequency of eating fish and seafood varies according to climate, age, sex, and personal needs and can range from once in awhile to more regularly, the standard being about once or twice per week in a temperate climate.

The kinds of fish and seafood recommended are those with less fat and cholesterol and those that are most easily digestible, especially low fat, white-meat varieties. As a separate side dish, fresh fish is usually prepared in a small to moderate amount as a supplement to whole grains and vegetables, which still comprise the major volume of the meal. It may also be served in soups or stews and cooked with other foods. The varieties of white-meat fish recommended for occasional consumption include the following as examples:

Ocean varieties	*Freshwater Varieties*
Cod	Bass
Flounder	Carp
Haddock	Catfish
Halibut	Pike
Herring	Trout
Ocean trout	Whitefish
Perch	Other varieties of white-
Scrod	meat, freshwater fish
Shad	
Smelt	*Dried Fish*
Sole	Bonito flakes (dried bonita,
Other varieties of white-	freshly shredded)
meat fish	Chirimen iriko (very small
	dried fish)
	Dried white-meat fish

Note: Shellfish such as lobster, crab meat, and shrimp are best limited or avoided for optimum health as they are high in cholesterol.

Broiled or Grilled White-meat Fish

To boil or grill fish, marinate in a mixture of equal parts water and tamari soy sauce and a few drops or fresh ginger juice for 1 hour or simply sprinkle with freshly squeezed lemon juice and a few drops of tamari soy sauce. Broil or grill until tender and flaky. Remove and serve with a garnish and grated daikon.

Steamed or Boiled White-meat Fish

Marinate as above or place plain fish in a steamer basket or saucepan. Steam or boil until tender and flaky. Remove and serve with a garnish and grated daikon.

Steamed Haddock

1½ lb haddock, washed and cut into 4–5 equal-sized pieces
4–5 broccoli flowerettes
¼ cup carrots, sliced in thick matchsticks or flower shapes
water
3 lemon slices for garnish
1 cup tamari-ginger dip sauce

Place the haddock in a ceramic bowl. Attractively arrange the broccoli flowerettes and carrots in the bowl with the haddock. Set the bowl down inside a pot with about 1/2 inch of water in the pot. Cover the pot and bring the water to a boil. Steam for several minutes until the haddock is tender and the vegetables are brightly colored and tender. Remove, garnish with lemon slices, and serve with the tamari-ginger dip sauce.

Tamari-Ginger Dip Sauce

⅛ tsp grated ginger
1 Tbsp tamari soy sauce
2 Tbsp water

Mix ingredients and heat up. Serve in a small cup or bowl.

Baked Sole with Rice

2–3 lb fresh fillet of sole
4 cups brown rice, pressure-cooked or boiled
dark sesame oil
1 cup onions, diced
½ cup celery, diced
¼ cup parsley, chopped
½ cup tamari soy sauce
½ cup water
1 tsp fresh grated ginger
several lemon wedges

Heat a small amount of dark sesame oil in a skillet. Sauté onions and celery for 2 to 3 minutes. Place sautéed vegetables in a bowl with rice and parsley and mix well. Transfer mixture to a casserole dish.

Mix tamari soy sauce, water, and ginger together. Place sole in a shallow bowl or dish and pour tamari-water-ginger mixture over it. Let sole marinate for 30 to 45 minutes. Place marinated sole evenly on top of rice in casserole dish. Cover casserole and bake at 350°F for approximately 30 minutes or until the sole becomes tender. Remove casserole cover and bake another 5 minutes. Sprinkle a little chopped parsley over the sole and serve with several lemon wedges for garnish.

Koi-koku (Carp-Burdock-Miso Soup)

> **1 small fresh carp**
> **dark sesame oil (optional)**
> **burdock (same in weight as carp), shaved**
> **$\frac{1}{2}$–1 cup used bancha twigs, wrapped and tied tightly in a**
> **cheesecloth sack**
> **water**
> **puréed barley miso to taste**
> **$\frac{1}{2}$–1 Tbsp fresh grated ginger**
> **sliced scallions for garnish**

Ask the fish seller to carefully remove the gallbladder and the yellow bitter bone (thyroid) and leave the rest of the carp intact. This includes the head, fins, tail, and scales. Next ask him to cut the carp into chunks. He may even remove the eyes, if you wish. Wash the carp and set aside.

Place a small amount of dark sesame oil in a pressure cooker and heat up. Add the shaved burdock and sauté for 2 to 3 minutes. Place the cheesecloth sack filled with used bancha twigs on top of the burdock. The tea twigs will help to soften the hard bones of the carp. Do not use fresh unused twigs as they will make the soup taste very bitter. Set the carp on top of the burdock and twigs. Add enough water to cover the carp and burdock. Place the cover on the pressure cooker and bring up to pressure. Reduce the flame to medium-low and cook for 1 1/2 to 2 hours. Remove from the flame and allow the pressure to come down. Remove the cover, add enough puréed miso for a mild salt taste (1/2 to 1 teaspoon puréed barley miso per cup of soup), and add the ginger. Reduce the flame to low and simmer until the bones are soft. Place in serving bowls and garnish with sliced scallions.

Carp soup is very strong and is best eaten in small volume. One cup at a time daily for 2 to 3 days is sufficient in most cases. If taken in larger quantities, it may cause cravings for fruits, liquids, sweets, or other strong yin foods.

Carp soup can be stored in a tightly sealed glass jar in the refrigerator for about 5 to 7 days. However, if frozen, it loses freshness and energy.

If carp is not available, you may substitute freshwater trout. Have the insides removed and leave the rest of the trout intact. If burdock is not available, you may substitute carrots sliced in matchsticks. (Half burdock and half carrots can also be used.) If you use trout, the time needed for pressure cooking is reduced to 50 to 60 minutes. After seasoning with puréed miso and grated ginger, simmer for several more minutes on a low flame. Garnish and serve hot.

Fish and Vegetable Soup

> 1–1½ lbs white-meat fish (scrod, cod, haddock, sole, etc.)
> 1 strip kombu, 1–2 inches long, soaked and diced
> ½ cup onions, sliced in thick wedges
> ¼ cup celery, sliced on a thick diagonal
> ½ cup daikon, quartered and sliced in ¼-inch pieces
> 1 cup carrots, sliced in chunks
> 2 Tbsp burdock, quartered and sliced
> 4–5 cups water
> sea salt, tamari soy sauce, or puréed barley miso
> sliced scallions or parsley for garnish

Place the kombu in a pot and add the onions, celery, daikon, carrots, and burdock. Add the water and a small pinch of sea salt. Cover and bring to a boil. Reduce the flame to medium-low and simmer until the vegetables are soft and tender. Add the fish, cover, and reduce the flame to low. Simmer 4 to 5 minutes until the fish is done. Season with a small amount of sea salt, tamari soy sauce, or puréed barley miso for a mild salt taste. Simmer 5 to 10 minutes more if using sea salt, or 2 to 3 minutes if using tamari soy sauce or puréed miso. Garnish with sliced scallions or parsley and serve hot.

You may occasionally add a small amount of grated ginger at the end of cooking for a different flavor. Please feel free to use other ground or root vegetables instead of the ones listed above.

Clear Fish Soup

> 1–2 fillets of sole (or other white-meat fish)
> 1 cup wakame, soaked, stems removed, and cut into 1-inch slices
> 3 shiitake mushrooms, soaked and sliced
> 5–6 cups kombu stock (add shiitake soaking water)
> tamari soy sauce to taste
> 1 bunch watercress, previously boiled for 1 second

Bring wakame, shiitake, and kombu stock to a boil, turn the flame down, and simmer for a few minutes until the wakame and shiitake soften. Cut the fillets of sole into 1 1/2- to 2-inch pieces and add them to the soup with tamari soy sauce to taste. Simmer for 1 to 2 minutes or until the sole turns white. Ladle the soup into individual serving bowls and garnish with the watercress. Serves 6 to 8.

Condiments

A variety of condiments may be used, some daily and others occasionally. Small amounts may be used on grains, soups, vegetables, beans, and other dishes. Condiments allow everyone to freely adjust the taste and nutritional value of foods, and stimulate and contribute to better appetite and digestion. The most frequently used varieties include:

Main Condiments
Gomashio (a half-crushed mixture of roasted sesame seeds
   and roasted sea salt)
Sea vegetable powder
Sea vegetable powder with roasted sesame seeds
Tekka (selected root vegetables sautéed with dark sesame
   oil and seasoned with soybean, or Hatcho, miso)
Umeboshi plum (pickled plums)

Other Condiments
Cooked miso with scallions or onions
Nori condiment (nori cooked with tamari soy sauce)
Roasted sesame seeds
Shiso leaf powder
Shio *kombu* (kombu cooked with tamari soy sauce)
Green nori flakes
Brown rice vinegar (used mostly as a seasoning)
Umeboshi plum and raw scallions or onions
Umeboshi vinegar (used mostly as a seasoning)
Other traditionally used condiments (not highly stimulating
   ones)

Gomashio (Sesame Salt)

1 cup black sesame seeds, washed and drained
1 Tbsp sea salt

Place the sea salt in a hot skillet and dry roast several minutes
over a medium flame until it becomes shiny. Remove and grind
to a fine powder in a suribachi. Next, place the damp sesame
seeds in a heated skillet and dry roast over a medium-low
flame, stirring constantly with a wooden rice paddle. Shake the
skillet back and forth occasionally to evenly roast. When the
sesame seeds give off a nutty fragrance and begin popping, take
a sesame seed and crush it between your thumb and ring finger.
If it crushes easily, the sesame seeds are done. If not, roast them
a little longer. When the sesame seeds are done, place them in
the suribachi and slowly grind together with the sea salt. Con-

tinue grinding until the sesame seeds are about half crushed. Allow to cool and store in a tightly sealed glass container. Use moderately on grains, noodles, or vegetable dishes. Tan sesame seeds can be substituted for black sesame seeds for variety.

Sea Vegetable Powders

Take several pieces of kombu, wakame, or dulse and place them, unwashed, on a baking sheet. Roast in a 350°F oven for approximately 15 to 20 minutes, or until crispy and dark but not burnt, or place in a dry skillet and roast until crispy and dark. Remove and break the roasted sea vegetable into small pieces over a suribachi. Crush into a fine powder. Allow to cool and store in a tightly sealed glass container. Sprinkle lightly on grains, noodles, or vegetable dishes.

Sea Vegetable and Roasted Sesame Seed Powders

Roast one of the above sea vegetables as explained. After roasting, grind into a fine powder in a suribachi. Dry roast washed and drained tan sesame seeds as you would if making gomashio. When done, place the roasted sesame seeds in the suribachi and grind with the sea vegetable powder until the sesame seeds are about 50 percent crushed. Allow to cool and store in a tightly sealed glass container. Use as you would gomashio or roasted sea vegetable powders. The average proportion of sesame seeds to powdered sea vegetables can be about 60 percent to 40 percent.

Tekka

This condiment is made from minced burdock, lotus root, carrot, Hatcho miso, and dark sesame oil. Toward the end of cooking it is seasoned with ginger juice. It is cooked over a low flame in a cast iron skillet until the ingredients turn completely black. It can be purchased prepackaged in natural food stores. Use moderately on grains, noodles, or vegetable dishes.

Nori Condiment

5 sheets nori, unroasted
water
tamari soy sauce

Tear the nori into small squares and place in a saucepan. Add
water to just cover. Bring to a boil, cover, and reduce the flame
to low. Simmer until the nori becomes a smooth, thick paste.
Season with several drops of tamari soy sauce for a mild salt
taste and continue to cook until all liquid is gone. Allow to cool
and store in the refrigerator, in a tightly sealed glass container.
Eat with grains, noodles, or vegetable dishes. A small amount
of freshly grated ginger may be added at the end of cooking for
a special flavor.

Shio Kombu Condiment

2 strips kombu, 10–12 inches long, dusted off, soaked, and
    cubed
water
tamari soy sauce

Place the kombu in a pot and just cover with a mixture of half
water and half tamari soy sauce. Bring to a boil, cover, and
reduce the flame to medium-low. Simmer until the kombu is
soft and then cook off most of the remaining liquid. Only 2 or
3 pieces are eaten with the meal as this condiment is quite salty.
To prepare this as a side dish, not a condiment, reduce the content of tamari soy sauce considerably.

   Variations of this condiment can be made by adding dried
fish such as chirimen or chuba; thin matchstick pieces of ginger;
thinly sliced shiitake; or even barley malt or rice syrup for a
sweet condiment.

Miso Scallion Condiment

2 cups scallions, chopped (chop the roots very fine and sauté
    first)
1 Tbsp barley miso

1 tsp dark sesame oil
2 Tbsp water

Sauté the scallions in dark sesame oil for 2 to 3 minutes. Purée the miso in a suribachi with a small amount of water. Add miso to scallions and gently mix. Place on a low flame, cover, and cook for 5 to 10 minutes. Serve with grain, noodle, or vegetable dishes.

Instead of scallions, chives, carrot tops, green peppers, onions, or parsley may be used.

Shiso Nori Condiment

2 tsp shiso leaves, very finely chopped and dry-roasted
    2–3 minutes
2 Tbsp *aonori* (green nori flakes)
$\frac{1}{2}$ cup sesame seeds, roasted

Place the shiso in a suribachi and grind slightly. Add the sesame seeds and aonori and mix. Store in a sealed glass container. Sprinkle occasionally on grains, vegetables, or noodle dishes.

Wakame Condiment

1 cup wakame, soaked and sliced
2 Tbsp brown rice vinegar
2 Tbsp tamari soy sauce
2 Tbsp spring water (optional)
1 Tbsp sesame seeds, washed and roasted

Put the wakame into a pot. Add the brown rice vinegar and tamari soy sauce. Add 2 tablespoons of water, if desired, and bring to a boil. Cover, reduce the flame to low, and simmer until almost all the liquid has evaporated, about 10 to 20 minutes. Garnish with sesame seeds.

Pickles

A small amount of natural vegetable pickles can be eaten daily or often as a supplement to main dish. They stimulate appetite and help digestion. Some varieties—such as pickled daikon or *takuan*—can be bought prepackaged in natural food stores. Others—such as quick pickles—can be prepared at home. Certain varieties take just a few hours to prepare, while others require more time.

A wide variety of pickles are fine for regular use, including, salt, salt brine, bran, miso, tamari soy sauce, umeboshi vinegar, and others. Natural sauerkraut may also be used in small volume on an occasional basis. Below are the varieties of pickles recommended for use:

Regular Use	*Avoid (for optimum health)*
Rice bran pickles	Dill pickles
Brine pickles	Herb pickles
Miso bean pickles	Garlic pickles
Miso pickles	Spiced pickles
Pressed pickles	Vinegar pickles (commercial
Sauerkraut	apple cider vinegar or
Tamari soy sauce pickles	wine vinegar pickles)
Takuan pickles	
Amazaké pickles	

Umeboshi-Vegetable Pickles

Place 7 to 8 umeboshi plums in a glass jar and add 2 quarts of water. Shake well and allow to sit several hours until the water becomes pink. Place a variety of thinly sliced vegetables (red radish, daikon, carrots, onions, cauliflower flowerettes, broccoli flowerettes, red onions, cabbage, etc.) in the water. Cover the jar with clean, cotton cheesecloth and place in a cool place for 3 to 5 days. When done, remove, or if too salty, rinse quickly under cold water and serve.

Quick Tamari Soy Sauce-Vegetable Pickles

Slice a variety of root or ground vegetables into thin slices and place in a glass jar. Cover with a mixture of half water and half tamari soy sauce. Shake and cover the jar with clean, cotton cheesecloth. Allow to sit in a cool place for 2 to 3 hours. Remove and serve or if too salty, rinse quickly and serve.

Longer Tamari Soy Sauce-Vegetable Pickles

Prepare as above but only allow the vegetables to pickle in the tamari-water solution for 3 to 5 days. Remove, rinse, and serve.

Tamari-Onion Pickles

> 2 cups onions, sliced in thin half-moons, parboiled 30 seconds
> ½ cup shiitake mushrooms, sliced thin and boiled 10–15 minutes
> 1 cup water
> ½ cup tamari soy sauce
> 1 tsp brown rice or sweet rice vinegar
> 1 Tbsp barley malt or rice syrup

Allow the onions and shiitake to cool and then place in a quart glass jar. Pour a mixture of half water and half tamari soy sauce over the vegetables to cover them. Add the brown rice or sweet rice vinegar and barley malt or rice syrup. Cover then shake to mix. Allow to sit 2 to 3 days or up to 1 week. Remove, rinse, and serve.

Small onions may be pickled whole, either raw or parboiled for 1 to 2 minutes.

Cucumber Pickles

> 2–3 lbs pickling cucumbers, washed
> 10–12 cups water
> ¼–⅓ cup sea salt
> 3–4 sprigs of fresh or dry dill
> 1 large onion, halved then each half quartered

Combine the water and sea salt. Bring to a boil and simmer 2 to 3 minutes until the sea salt dissolves. Allow to cool. Place cucumbers, dill, and onion slices in a large glass jar or a ceramic crock. Pour the cooled salt-water over the vegetables. Allow to sit uncovered in a dark, cool place for 3 to 4 days. Cover and refrigerate. Let sit 2 to 3 more days. Cucumbers will keep about 1 month in the refrigerator.

Vegetables such as cauliflower, broccoli, daikon, carrots, red radishes, or watermelon rinds may also be pickled in the same manner.

Sauerkraut

5 lbs cabbage (white kraut cabbage is best), washed
¼–⅓ cup sea salt

Slice the cabbage very thin. Place the cabbage in a ceramic crock or wooden keg and add the sea salt. Mix thoroughly. Place a wooden lid or plate, that is slightly smaller than the crock, on top of the cabbage so that it fits down inside the crock. Place a heavy weight on top of the lid. Cover the top of the crock with a piece of cheesecloth.

After a day, water should cover the cabbage; if not, apply a heavier weight. Keep in a dark, cool place for about 2 weeks. Check the crock daily. If the mold forms on the top, skim and discard. If the mold is not removed, the sauerkraut will develop a moldy taste. The mold is not harmful as it results naturally from the fermentation process. It merely detracts from the taste. To serve, rinse under cold water and place in a serving dish.

Turnip-Kombu Pickles

3 medium-sized turnips, washed
1 strip kombu, 8–10 inches long, soaked
sea salt

Slice the turnips in half. Then slice each half into almost paper-thin half-moons. Sprinkle several pinches of sea salt on the bottom of a ceramic crock or wooden keg. Place the turnips in the crock, little by little, in layers. After each layer of turnips sprinkle a couple pinches of sea salt. Repeat until turnips are used up.

Place a wooden lid, or a plate small enough to set down inside the crock, on top of the turnips. Place a heavy weight such as a clean stone or brick on top of the lid. When the water level rises to the lid, drain off all the salty water. Remove the turnips.

Slice the kombu into very thin matchsticks and mix the kombu and turnips together and place back in the crock. Replace the disc and stone on top. Keep in a cool place for 1 or 2 days. When pickles are ready to eat, the liquid surrounding the turnips will thicken and become very slippery. This is how they should turn if correctly made.

They are now ready to eat. Refrigerate to store.

Daikon-Lemon Pickles

4 cups daikon, sliced in ⅛-inch-thick rounds or rectangles
5–6 matchstick-sized pieces of lemon rind
sea salt

Place daikon and lemon in a ceramic crock or wooden keg. Add a small amount of sea salt to create a mild salt taste. Mix thoroughly. Place a lid or plate on top of the daikon. Place a clean stone or brick on top of the lid to apply pressure. After 4 hours remove the lemon rind and discard.

When the water level reaches the lid or plate, place a lighter weight stone or brick on top. Keep in a cool place for 2 to 3 days.

Rinse and serve.

Pressed Quick Red Radish Pickles

2 cups red radish and their greens, sliced thin
1–2 Tbsp umeboshi vinegar

Place the red radish, greens, and umeboshi vinegar in a pickle press and mix well. Secure the top on the press and screw down to apply pressure. Let sit for 2 to 3 days. Remove, rinse, and serve.

Brine Pickles

Boil 3 to 4 cups of water together with 1 teaspoon of sea salt until the sea salt is completely dissolved. Allow to cool completely. Place a 3-inch piece of kombu in a jar and pour the cool salt brine over it. Place thin slices of root or ground vegetables such as carrots, daikon, radishes, onions, broccoli, cauliflower, cucumber, and others in the water. Cover the jar with clean, cotton cheesecloth and let sit in a slightly cool and dark place for 3 days (not the refrigerator). These pickles are best stored in the refrigerator.

Seasonings

A variety of naturally processed seasonings are fine for regular use. Unrefined sea salt is used regularly in cooking whole grains, beans, and many vegetables. Tamari soy sauce, miso, and umeboshi plums, which have been salted and pickled, are also used frequently, but in general, the use of seasonings is best kept moderate. Rather than using them to add a salty flavor to your dishes, it is better to use them to bring forth the natural light sweetness of the whole grains, vegetables, beans, and sea vegetables, and other ingredients you are cooking with. The use of sea salt is a highly individual matter and is based on factors such as age, sex, activity, and climate in which we are living.

The following seasonings are used most often in macrobiotic cooking:

Regular Use
Miso, especially barley
  (mugi) and soybean
  (Hatcho)
Tamari soy sauce
Unrefined white sea salt

Occasional Use
Ginger
Horseradish
Mirin

Rice vinegar
Umeboshi vinegar
Umeboshi plum or paste
Sesame oil (dark)

Avoid (for optimum health)
All commercial seasonings
All stimulating and aromatic
  spices and herbs
All irradiated spices and herbs

Beverages

A variety of natural beverages can be included for daily, regular, or occasional consumption. The frequency and amount of beverage intake vary according to the individual's personal condition and needs as well as the climate, season, and other environmental factors. Generally, it is advisable to drink comfortably and when thirsty and to avoid icy cold drinks. The following beverages are used most often in the practice of macrobiotics:

Regular Use
Bancha tea (kukicha)
Bancha stem tea
Roasted barley tea
Roasted brown rice tea
Natural spring water
 (suitable for daily use)
High quality natural well
 water

Occasional Use
Grain coffee (100 percent
 roasted cereal grains)
Sweet vegetable broth
Dandelion tea
Kombu tea
Umeboshi tea
Mu tea
Freshly squeezed carrot juice
 (if desired, about 2 cups
 per week)

Infrequent Use
Green leaf tea
Green magma
Vegetable juice
Northern climate fruit juice
Beer (natural quality)
Saké (natural quality)
Wine (natural quality)

Avoid (for Optimum Health)
Distilled water
Coffee
Cold or ice drinks
Hard liquor
Aromatic herbal tea
Mineral water and all
 bubbling waters
Chemically colored tea
Stimulant beverages
Sugared drinks
Tap water
Artificial, chemically treated
 beverages
Tropical fruit juices

Bancha Twig Tea (Kukicha)

Place 1 tablespoon of bancha twigs in 1 quart of water and bring to a boil. Reduce the flame to low. Simmer 1 to 3 minutes for a mild taste or up to 15 minutes for a stronger tea. Drink while hot.

Bancha Stem Tea

Bancha stem tea is made entirely of twigs and contains no leaves. It is prepared in the same manner as kukicha but requires a slightly longer cooking time.

Roasted Grain Tea

Dry roast about 1/2 cup of washed barley or brown rice in a skillet until golden yellow, stirring constantly to prevent burning. Place the roasted grains in a quart of water and bring to a boil. Reduce the flame to low and simmer for about 15 to 20 minutes. Drink while hot.

Roasted Barley Tea

You may purchase prepackaged, unhulled, roasted barley tea in most natural food stores. Place 1 tablespoon of roasted barley in a quart of water and bring to a boil. Reduce the flame to low and simmer 1 to 3 minutes for a mild tea or up to 10 minutes for a stronger flavored beverage. Drink while hot or room temperature in hotter weather.

Umeboshi Tea

Umeboshi tea has a cooling effect in hot weather and helps to replace mineral salts which are lost through perspiration.

Remove umeboshi meat from the pits of 2 to 3 umeboshi plums and add to 1 quart of water. Bring to a boil, reduce the flame, and simmer about 1/2 hour.

Sweet Vegetable Drink

$\frac{1}{2}$ cup carrots, diced
$\frac{1}{2}$ cup onions, diced
$\frac{1}{2}$ cup winter squash, sliced very thin
$\frac{1}{2}$ cup green cabbage, sliced very thin
2 quarts water

Place all ingredients in a pot, cover, and bring to a boil. Reduce the flame to low and simmer for 10 to 15 minutes. Remove from the flame and strain the sweet broth. Drink 1 cup or so. Store in a glass jar in the refrigerator and heat up as needed. Save the cooked vegetables from making the broth and use in soups.

Apple Juice or Cider

If one's condition is generally good, an occasional glass of apple cider or juice may be enjoyed. In the summer, apple juice can be served cool or lightly chilled, but not icy cold, as this has a paralyzing effect on the digestive tract. In cool weather, heat the apple cider or juice and drink it hot. This can help neutralize an overly yang condition resulting from the intake of too much salt.

Homemade Amazaké

Amazaké is a natural sweetener, dessert, or sweet drink made from fermented sweet rice or regular brown rice. It can be used as a sweetener for cookies, cakes, breads, pancakes, and donuts. Amazaké can also be blended. Serve it hot or cool.

4 cups brown rice or regular brown rice
8 cups water
1 cup *koji*
pinch of sea salt

Wash the rice, drain, and soak overnight in 8 cups of water. Place the rice in a pressure cooker. Bring to pressure, reduce the flame to medium-low, and simmer for 20 minutes. Turn off the flame and let the rice sit in the pressure cooker for 45 minutes.

Allow to cool. When the rice is cool enough, handle by hand and mix the koji in. Place the rice and koji in a glass bowl and keep in a warm place for 4 to 8 hours (no longer than 8 hours). Several times, mix the rice and koji to help the koji melt. Place a pinch of sea salt and the rice in a pot and bring to a boil. As soon as bubbles come to the surface, turn off the flame. Allow to cool. Place the rice in a glass bowl or jar and refrigerate.

To keep for a long time, amazaké can be cooked over a low flame until it becomes slightly brown.

When using as a sweetener either add as is to pastries, or blend to make it smooth.

For a beverage, dilute with a little water and blend until thick and creamy.

For Further Reading

Colbin, Annemarie. *Food and Healing*. New York: Ballantine, 1986.

Esko, Edward and Wendy. *Macrobiotic Cooking for Everyone*. Tokyo and New York: Japan Publications, Inc., 1980.

Esko, Wendy. *Aveline Kushi's Introducing Macrobiotic Cooking*. Tokyo and New York: Japan Publications, Inc., 1987.

Kushi, Aveline, and Wendy Esko. *The ·Changing Seasons Macrobiotic Cookbook*. Wayne, N.J.: Avery Publishing Group, 1983.

Kushi, Michio, and Alex Jack. *The Cancer Prevention Diet*. New York: St. Martin's Press, 1983.

———. *Diet for a Strong Heart*. New York: St. Martin's Press, 1984.

Kushi, Michio and Aveline, with Alex Jack. *Macrobiotic Diet*. Tokyo and New York: Japan Publications, Inc., 1985.

Pritikin, Nathan. *Diet for Runners*. New York: Simon and Schuster, Inc., 1985.

Sattilaro, Anthony, M.D., with Tom Monte. *Recalled by Life: The Story of My Recovery from Cancer*. Boston: Houghton-Mifflin, 1982.

———. *Living Well Naturally*. Boston: Houghton-Mifflin, 1984.

Tara, William. *Macrobiotics and Human Behavior*. Tokyo and New York: Japan Publications, Inc., 1985.

Turner, Kristina. *The Self-Healing Cookbook*. Grass Valley, Calif.: Earthtones Press, 1989.

For more information on macrobiotics:

Contact:

The Kushi Institute
P.O. Box 7
Becket, Mass. 01223
413–623–5742

List of Recipes

Index

264